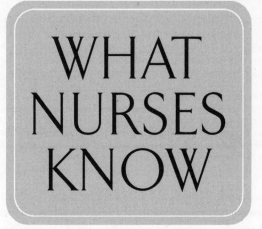

# WHAT NURSES KNOW

## AND DOCTORS DON'T HAVE TIME TO TELL YOU

Patricia Carroll, R.N.

A Perigee Book

The information in this book is not intended as a substitute for the advice of physicians or other qualified health professionals. It is not intended to be prescriptive with references to any specific ailment or condition, or to the general health of the reader, but rather a description of one approach to fostering health and wellness. The reader is advised to consult with his or her physician before undertaking any of the practices contained in this book. The reader should also continue to consult regularly with his or her physician in matters relating to his or her health, particularly in respect to any symptom that may require diagnosis or medical treatment. Neither the author nor the publisher shall be liable or responsible for any loss, injury, or damage allegedly arising from the use of any information contained in this book.

A Perigee Book
Published by The Berkley Publishing Group
A division of Penguin Group (USA) Inc.
375 Hudson Street
New York, New York 10014

Perigee trade paperback edition: June 2004

Visit our website at www.penguin.com

Library of Congress Cataloging-in-Publication Data

Carroll, Patricia.
What nurses know and doctors don't have time to tell you / Patricia Carroll.—
Perigee trade pbk. ed.
p. cm.
Includes bibliographical references.
ISBN 0-399-52957-8
1. Nursing. 2. Nurse and patient. 3. Nursing—Practice. 4. Nurses—Attitudes.
5. Nurse and physician. I. Title

RT41.C2916 2004
610.73—dc22

Printed in the United States of America

10 9 8 7 6 5 4

# CONTENTS

## 2. Treating and Preventing Injuries

## 3. Choosing and Using Medicines Wisely

## 4. You and the Health Care System

# 5. MEDICAL TESTS AND SAME-DAY SURGERY

# ACKNOWLEDGMENTS

Any serious writer will tell you that while one name may appear on the cover, an extended family shares in shaping the book before we send it off on its own and into your hands. It's not often that you get to hold a dream in your hand, but this book is a dream that started when I was in the first grade and would get my friends together to write and illustrate our own little books; it has now grown into a book that I hope will help far more people than I could ever personally care for as a bedside nurse.

John Duff, my publisher, understood from the very beginning that a registered nurse had a unique perspective on health and a wealth of practical knowledge to share. He has the patience of Job, and I could not ask for more from a publisher. I tell Katie McHugh, who edited this manuscript, that I owe her forever for her incredibly skilled work on this project and for providing the critically important feedback that made this book so much better because of her thoughtful contributions and suggestions. (Writers tend to be terrified of editors because we don't know if they will understand our point of view and keep our quirky personalities in our works. Katie "got it" in spades. Whew!)

To my non-nurse friends and professional colleagues who have taught me so much and supported me in so many ways over the years: Carl Wiezalis, Karen Milikowski, David Howell, Beth

Richards, Jeff McGill, Steve Herweck, Glenn Hawkes, Jeff Mac-Donald, Judy Linn, Denise Dickerson, Deepu Advani, Marcia Proto, Louis Blumenfeld, Anthony DeWitt, Sandi Gangell, Harriet Unger, and Elaine Lisitano.

To the doctors who somehow found the time to tell me things and helped me learn: Thomas Manger, who gave the manuscript two thumbs up and wants all of his patients to read it; Eric Silverstein, who keeps me on my toes; Matthew Saidel, who I took a chance on when he started private practice and am still with him "more than twenty" years later; Steve Balloch, who makes me smile; Mark O'Malley, who keeps me in line; and the late Bruce Farrell, who taught me that sometimes it's best when a suffering patient dies.

And, to the men and women who have walked in the same white shoes that I have, and know things that only nurses know, and have always been so generous in sharing their time and knowledge with me: Barbara Acello, Norma Amsterdam, Cynthia Bautista, Ellen Boyda, Linda Carl, Tracy Evans, Pat Greenberg, Wendie Howland, Suzanne Hall Johnson, Vincent Maher, Richard Nadan, Leslie Nicoll, Sarah Perry, Regina Pilatti, Linda Smith, Gail Talbott, Wilson Tay, Clare Thompson, Diane Wadsworth, Nancy Zeidel, and the nurse who I think is the sister I never had, Teri Mills.

And finally, to the help from Kirby, Mel, and Paulie—you know who you are.

# DEDICATION

This is for my husband. When we shared our vows in 1984, I had no idea how much he really meant the parts that said, ". . . for worse, . . . for poorer, . . . for sickness, . . . and to love, honor, and cherish." This book simply wouldn't have happened without his unconditional support. I am truly blessed to have someone who shares my dreams, celebrates my joys, and cushions my pain.

When we met, I was still in nursing school. He had *some* idea what he was getting himself into, but neither of us realized our path would lead us to doing the volunteer work necessary to establish a free health clinic that started as one for the homeless, and with the growing health care crisis has grown to include anyone in our community who needs health care and can't afford it. His willingness to learn about nursing, help out when we need it, and his generosity and genuine respect for the people we serve is an inspiration to everyone he works with.

What this nurse knows is that she couldn't have done it (any of it) alone.

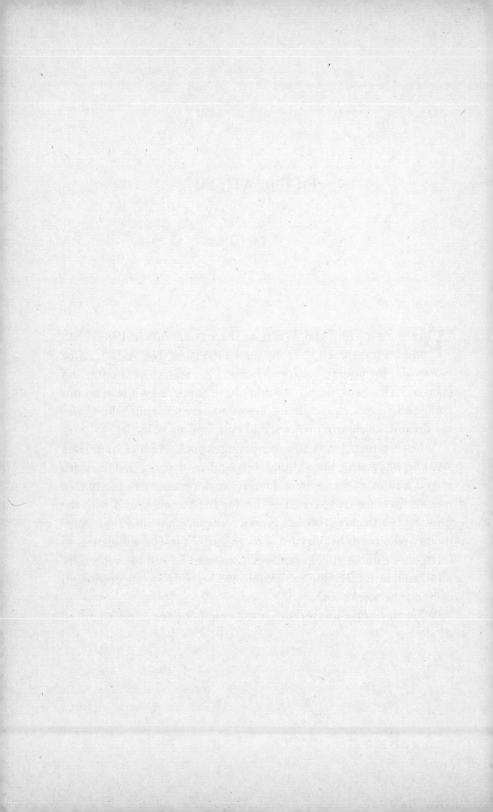

# INTRODUCTION

Welcome to my world—the world of the nurse. Nurses have a different perspective on providing care compared with physicians, and it starts with the definition of our professions. Physicians diagnose and treat *illness*. Nurses, on the other hand, diagnose and treat the *human response to illness*. From day one, a physician's education is focused on the disease, illness, or injury, while a nurse's education is focused on how that same disease, illness, or injury affects the person.

That doesn't mean this book is anti-physician or that I don't like physicians! I work with them almost every day, and we are all members of a team whose ultimate interest is the best care for the patient. Professionally, we come from different perspectives, that's all.

With that philosophy in mind, this book is different from other "self-care" or "medical advisor" books. Instead of organizing things by diagnosis (so the book is hard to use unless you can diagnose yourself correctly first), I'll discuss signs and symptoms in relation to how you feel, and what you can do to feel better. That also means no laundry lists of tests that may or may not be done because each person should be treated as an individual, based on his or her unique signs, symptoms, and health history. I also won't take a lot of time explaining all the structures and functions of your body;

there are plenty of resources out there if you want to learn that. Where needed, I'll fill you in to enhance your understanding.

If you do have something serious such as a brain tumor or cancer, that's the kind of situation in which your doctor will have time to tell you about it. Self-care is not the place to start! So this book covers the basics—the most common conditions. I'll never forget the first doctor who took time to explain things to me when I was a student, and got a kick out of my "Gee whiz!" enthusiasm. His name was Dr. Bruce Farrell, and he taught me one of the rules of medicine you never want to forget: If you hear hoof beats, look for horses, not zebras. As a nursing student or instructor, we're so busy teaching or studying and learning about rare and exotic conditions that we think they're everywhere. More often than not, the cause is much more common and benign. In this book, we'll cover horses, not zebras.

That said, and to keep the book from being thousands of pages long, I have taken some shortcuts.

- ■ "Call the doctor," or "Talk to your doctor." I am on a campaign to change this mind-set. I prefer "Call your *health care provider*," or "Talk to your *health care provider*." Today and for the foreseeable future, primary care will no be provided exclusively by physicians. Nurse practitioners and physician assistants are playing a greater role in health care. So, in this book, unless there is a discussion that specifically needs to be addressed by a physician, you'll see the letters "HCP" for health care provider and "PCP" for primary care practitioner. That means the professional practitioner you see for your regular primary care—physician or not.
- ■ I use "call 911" as shorthand for "call your local emergency rescue services." If your community does not have a 911 system, follow local instructions for how to summon an ambulance (and be sure those instructions are on every phone in your house).

■ Another abbreviation I use is "OTC" for over-the-counter
medicines you can buy without a prescription.

Other important information you'll need to know includes:

■ Recommendations in this book are for healthy adults. They do
not necessarily apply to children under the age of about 16. If
you have a chronic illness such as diabetes or asthma or HIV,
you may need to follow different instructions for care. If you
have any question about how your preexisting condition or
medicines you take every day might affect one of the topics
covered in this book, check with your HCP.
■ Never stop taking medicine or abandon the plan of care prescribed for you based solely on what you read in this book.
Instead, use this book as a tool to help you prepare questions for your HCP if your plan and the recommendations
here are very different. Feel free to send me an e-mail at
askpat@whatnursesknow.com if you need more information
about a particular topic. While I can't provide personal advice without examining you, I'll do what I can to answer
your questions or suggest references or Web sites.

Suggestions about when to call your HCP are specific to the topic
being discussed. Of course, you should call your HCP any time you
have concerns about your health and symptoms you're having.

## ■ 1 ■

# TREATING
# SYMPTOMS

# ▪ HEAD CASES ▪

## HEADACHES

### NURSE'S NOTE

So you've got a headache? Join the club. Ninety percent of men and 95% percent of women have at least one headache a year. Some people are more susceptible to having headaches—and then there are carriers, who inevitably cause headaches in others!

Very few headaches are caused by something serious such as a brain hemorrhage, infection, or brain tumor.

### GET THEE TO THE ER

You need to call 911 for a ride to the ER if you have:

- A severe headache that came on suddenly. Some people describe these headaches as feeling like a "bolt of lightning" or a "thunderclap."
- A bad headache and a stiff neck, and normal light hurts your eyes.
- A headache accompanied by numbness, tingling, weakness, trouble speaking, or droopiness on one side of your face.

■ A headache after you were knocked unconscious or you can't recall what happened.

Headaches are one of the top two symptoms of people who come to the ER because they want drugs, not because they are really sick. If you go to the ER with a headache and feel like you're getting the third degree, don't take it personally.

## CALL YOUR HEALTH CARE PROVIDER

■ If you usually have headaches, but this one is different in that it's lasting longer, is in a different spot or has different symptoms associated with it.

■ If you've taken prescribed headache medication, but it's not working.

■ If you have the same type of headache a few times a week, and you haven't talked to your HCP about it.

■ If you're missing work or school or are unable to carry out normal activities because of your headache(s).

■ If you have a headache and also notice a change in your ability to taste, hear, or smell.

■ If the headaches started after you began taking a new prescription or OTC medicine.

■ If you can't figure out why you're having a headache, but it is not severe and doesn't occur with other symptoms that require a trip to the ER.

## COMMON TYPES OF HEADACHES

### Tension headache.

Approximately seventy-five percent of all headaches are tension headaches. They're usually a steady ache caused by muscle tension in the scalp, neck, and face. You might feel like your head is in a vise or that there's a band squeezing your head. Tension headaches come and go (sometimes daily), do not come on suddenly, and are not disabling. Annoying, yes. Disabling, no. People rarely wake up with a tension headache. Instead you get them at the end of a long, stressful day, particularly if you haven't gotten much sleep and haven't had time to eat.

How you feel:
- Vice-like band around the head
- Comes on gradually during the day
- May also have neck and upper back pain

Nurse's order:
- OTC pain reliever

**Migraine.**
About one person in a hundred will have at least one migraine headache. A migraine is a specific diagnosis, not a catchall term to describe any bad headache. Three out of four people with true migraines are women. About 60% of the time, the pain is severe, on one side of the head, and is throbbing or pounding. A migraine makes you want to crawl into a very dark, quiet place because light and noise make the pain even worse. If you are having a true migraine, you may be sick to your stomach and may even vomit.

One in five people with migraines will have an aura—typically, flashing or bright lights that move across the field of vision. Some people may experience a partial loss of vision in one eye. Migraines may happen once or twice and can last for a few days, but they don't go away and come back daily.

How you feel:
- Pounding or throbbing pain, usually on one side of your head
- Pain often accompanied by nausea or vomiting

Other indicators:
- Might see flashing lights before the pain starts

Nurse's order:
- OTC pain reliever with caffeine
- Prescription medication to take at the first sign of the beginning of a migraine attack

**Cluster headache.**
This type of headache got its name because it comes in patterns or groups called clusters. Unlike people with migraines, who don't want to move, people with cluster headaches may pace or rock because the pain is so bad. These headaches can awaken you in the middle of the night—often at about the same time—over a few weeks. Then the headaches can go away for months or years. Only 1% of people have cluster headaches, and 85% occur in men. Cluster headaches have very typical characteristics, but it may be difficult to get to an HCP while one is occurring to get an "official" diagnosis.

How you feel:
- Severe pain, often described as feeling "like a hot poker in the eye"
- Pain often awakens you from sleep
- Pain occurs frequently for a period of time, then may go away for months or years

Other indicators:
- Eye is often tearing and red on the same side as where the pain occurs and nose may be plugged

Nurse's order:
- Prescription for pain medication from your HCP

## TECHNICALLY SPEAKING . . .

A headache does not mean your brain hurts because the brain has no pain sensors. Instead, you feel impulses from muscles, nerves, and blood vessels inside and outside the skull.

## ? Frequently Asked Questions

Q. *What causes migraines?*
A. There is some debate about this, but migraines are related to changes in the blood flow to the brain—either too much or too little blood flows in response to certain triggers that can range from foods to weather changes and even flickering lights.

Q. *Can substances in foods and drinks cause headaches?*
A. Absolutely. Many people can get a migraine after being exposed to sulfites, found in many wines, and once used in salad bars to keep the produce looking fresh. MSG is another culprit, as are food preservatives containing nitrates or nitrites, such as the sodium nitrite found in hot dogs. A headache diary can help you pinpoint your headache triggers.

Q. *Do headaches run in families?*
A. Migraines do; cluster headaches do not. However, if there is a lot of turmoil in a family, people can "learn" to have headaches if it gets them out of tense situations. In that case, headaches run in families behaviorally, but not genetically.

## NURSE'S WISDOM

- With a tension headache, you're less likely to be able to point to where it hurts with one finger than with other types of headaches.
- Any enteric-coated medicine (such as coated aspirin) will take longer to work because it won't break down until it leaves the stomach.
- Lie down with a scented eye pillow over your eyes. The pillow will block out light, and the scent (of your choosing) can be very relaxing. Eye pillows filled with flaxseed can be chilled in the freezer. I use the ones from It's My Nature (888-445-5051)

## Did You Know?

A study of people having chronic tension headaches (more than 15 a month) discovered that combining an antidepressant drug with stress management provided better relief than either treatment alone. In this research, patients were taught home management of stress, such as muscle relaxation, problem-solving techniques, coping skills, and using audiotapes as stress-management tools. Not as many pain relievers were needed because headaches were fewer and less severe.

because they use the principles of herbal medicine and have made different eye pillows containing different herbs based on whether you need to reduce stress, clear your nose, or rest your eyes after too much computer time.

■ If you have chronic headaches and are under the care of a specialist, ask for a note you can carry with you in case you need to go to the ER. The note will help establish your diagnosis and speed your care.

■ Do you wake up with a headache most mornings? Do you drink a lot of coffee or soda? If so, your morning headache may be due to caffeine withdrawal. If it goes away after that first cup in the morning, you can make your own diagnosis.

■ Drank too much alcohol the night before? Even if you're queasy, eat something because low blood sugar worsens the headache. Try honey on toast or crackers, these complex carbohydrates will help your liver get rid of the alcohol. Stay away from acetaminophen, which can stress an already overworked liver. And drink plenty of fluids as dehydration is one of the main causes of hangover symptoms.

■ Headache pain is real. Don't stand for an HCP who doesn't take your pain seriously "just because it's stress." Pain is what you tell us it is, and pain specialists have many tools at their disposal for you.

- If you're not getting relief from the remedies discussed here, mention your headaches to your dentist. Sometimes headaches can be related to what's commonly called TMJ, a disorder of the temporomandibular (TEMM-pour-oh-man-DIBB-you-lar) joint—the place where your lower jaw connects to your skull—or teeth grinding.

## SELF-CARE

Keep a headache diary. Your headache may be related to a particular food, time of day, situation, the weather, and, for women, the time in the menstrual cycle.

### Tension headache:
- Try the OTC pain reliever you like best.
- Avoid multisymptom remedies if you have a simple tension headache. Why take an antihistamine or decongestant if you don't need it?
- Put a heat or cold pack—whichever works best for you—across your forehead and at the base of your skull.
- Take a hot shower and let the water beat down on your upper neck and shoulders to relax the muscle spasms that can trigger headaches.
- Use aromatherapy such as an eye pillow, candle, or other scent to ease your mood. (I have coconut candle I light when I need to think about sitting on the beach in St. Thomas drinking a piña colada.)

### Migraine:
- Add caffeine to your pain medicine, which can help relieve migraine pain.
- If you think you are having true migraines, be sure to see your HCP for a work-up and clear diagnosis. Prescription drugs are available to prevent and treat the early phase of a migraine *before* the pain is disabling.

■ Go to a dark, quiet place if you are having a migraine headache. Unplug the phone.

**Everyday headaches:**
■ Don't starve. Low blood sugar can cause a splitting headache.
■ Try not to get drunk. The first drink always goes down fastest, so make it club soda or sparkling water. Drink one glass of water after every alcoholic drink.
■ Be sure to drink plenty of nonalcoholic fluids, particularly when it is hot outside. Dehydration can cause headaches, too.

## PAIN REMEDIES

One of the saddest experiences for me working in the ER was when, typically, a teenaged girl would come in after having taken an overdose of pain medicine—not necessarily to harm herself, but to "send a message" to someone with whom she was angry. "After all," these young women thought, "it's only headache medicine!" They had no idea that overdoses of acetaminophen can cause liver damage, and aspirin can cause bleeding and severe chemical abnormalities.

The maximum recommended dose of acetaminophen is 4,000 milligrams per day; yet people with liver damage took a median dose of 5,000 milligrams per day. These are fine medicines, but like any drug, you can't simply take extra doses without potentially serious consequences.

Reading labels is absolutely essential when choosing a pain medicine. Acetaminophen is used in hundreds of remedies, not just pain medicines. If you are particularly sensitive to caffeine, you may want to avoid the pain relievers that include caffeine. And, just because a product says "Tylenol" on the label doesn't mean it contains acetaminophen. In the future, other pain medicine brand names may be used as a product name for drugs that do not contain the pain medicine.

### Acetaminophen.

This is the active ingredient in Tylenol, a very popular OTC pain remedy. It is more gentle on the stomach than the other pain medicines. It has less anti-inflammatory properties than the other OTC pain medicines. However, it can be toxic to the liver.

### Acetaminophen/Aspirin/Caffeine.

This combination has been approved for use OTC to treat migraine pain in addition to other types of pain. Research shows that combining pain medicines from different categories can enhance pain relief and adding caffeine can relieve headache pain 40% better than taking the same medicine without caffeine.

### Aspirin.

This drug has been used for over a hundred years. It suppresses the body's pain messages to the brain and reduces the inflammation and swelling that often causes pain. Aspirin's most common side effect is stomach irritation; coated aspirin that dissolves in the intestine and not the stomach can protect the stomach, but the drug will not get into the body as quickly if you have a splitting headache.

### Aspirin/Caffeine.

Caffeine enhances the absorption of aspirin from the stomach when they're taken together for headache pain in particular, and taking this combination allows you to take lower doses of aspirin to get the same pain relief, lessening the chance of stomach irritation.

### Ibuprofen, Ketoprofen, Naproxen.

These are all nonsteroidal anti-inflammatory drugs, or NSAIDS (EN-seds). In addition to relieving pain and inflammation, these drugs are particularly effective in relieving menstrual cramps because of the way they work in the body to reduce prostaglandin, a hormone that accentuates inflammation and pain. No research shows one of these three drugs to be superior to the others; you'll need to see if one works better for you.

## ✚ When to Consider

- To treat mild to moderate pain.
- Some of these medicines will also reduce inflammation and swelling.

## 🚫 Do Not Use

- Do not take acetaminophen if you have liver disease.
- Do not take acetaminophen if you drink more than three alcoholic beverages a day.
- Do not take aspirin if you are taking prescription anticoagulants (blood thinners).
- Use caution with aspirin and NSAIDS if you've had a bleeding stomach ulcer.
- Use caution taking NSAIDS if you are taking medicine to lower your blood pressure; the interaction can lessen the effectiveness of the blood pressure drug(s).

## LISTEN UP!

- If you are having the worst headache you have ever had, and it came out of nowhere, go to the ER by ambulance.
- As tempting as it may be, do not take more than the recommended dose of any headache medicine. If you can't get relief from self-care call your HCP or go to the ER.
- If everybody in the home has a headache at once and no one is sick, you may have a carbon monoxide leak. Get out of the area and call the fire department to check carbon monoxide levels.

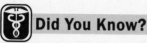

## Did You Know?

Caffeine boosts the effectiveness of pain relief when used with aspirin or acetaminophen, or with both in combination. To give you an idea of how much caffeine we're talking about, here are some comparisons:

| CAFFEINE SOURCE | AMOUNT IN MILLIGRAMS |
| --- | --- |
| Excedrin | 65 mg/tablet, 130 mg per dose |
| Anacin | 32 mg/tablet, 64 mg per dose |
| Brewed coffee, 8 oz | 135 mg |
| Diet Coke, 12 oz | 45 mg |
| Mountain Dew, 12 oz | 54 mg |
| No-Doz | 100 mg/tablet |
| Vivarin | 200 mg/tablet |

The average American consumes about 200–300 mg of caffeine per day, mostly from coffee.

# EARACHES AND HEARING LOSS

## NURSE'S NOTE

The most common ear problem is ear pain, usually caused by infection; fullness or pressure in the ear; and changes in hearing, which can include ringing in the ears, muffled sounds, or gradual hearing loss.

Earwax buildup is one of the most common causes of hearing loss. The most common cause of wax blockage? Attempts to clean the ear with cotton swabs or twisted washcloths that drive the wax too deep in the ear.

## GET THEE TO THE ER

Ear problems rarely need emergency treatment. However, you need to go to the ER if:

- You have severe ear pain.
- Your sudden hearing loss or change is associated with other symptoms such as a severe headache (see page 3) or vertigo (see page 73).

## CALL YOUR HEALTH CARE PROVIDER

- If ear pain persists or increases despite self-care, and you have a fever.
- If you have drainage from the ear that looks like blood and/or pus.
- If you have an earwax buildup that doesn't respond to self-care.
- If moderate pain persists for four or five days.
- If there is redness, swelling, or tenderness when you touch the bone behind your ear.
- If ringing in your ear(s) doesn't go away on its own within about 24 hours.

## COMMON TYPES OF EARACHES

### Ear infection.

There are two main types of ear infections: in the outer ear canal and in the middle ear.

An outer ear infection (also called swimmer's ear) is an inflammation with or without infection occurring in the outer ear canal—the part of the ear leading from the eardrum to the opening on the side of the head.

How you feel:
- Pain in outer ear that usually gets worse if you tug on the ear
- May be some hearing loss

Other indicators:
- Discharge from ear may be present
- Usually not sick
- Skin in ear canal may crack or flake due to chronic moisture

Nurse's order:
- Put a few drops of hydrogen peroxide in the ear, followed by a few drops of rubbing alcohol, to dry the ear canal. Use a dropper; never a cotton swab.
- Use antibiotic ear drops if your HCP determines an infection is present

## Middle ear infection or *otitis media* (oh-TY-tis MEE-dee-uh)

This is a bacterial or viral infection in the middle ear behind the eardrum. Pain comes from a bulging eardrum when fluid and pus are trapped behind it.

How you feel:
- Mild to severe pain deep in the ear
- Hearing may be muffled

Other indicators:
- May feel sick and have a fever
- Discharge is rare, unless eardrum ruptures

Nurse's order:
- OTC pain reliever
- Prescription to treat infection if indicated after an exam by your HCP

## Airplane ears.

This condition is caused by pressure buildup in the middle ear (see page 19).

How you feel:
- Pressure or fullness in the ears, and some ear pain
- Hearing loss and ringing in the ears possible

Nurse's order:
- OTC decongestants

## Earwax buildup.

Earwax is a thick liquid that normally coats the outer ear canal to trap particles and protect the eardrum. The wax normally drains out of the ear. Sometimes, though, it becomes dry and packed, particularly if you have poked in your ear with cotton swabs, your finger, or other small instruments.

How you feel:
- Hearing loss often the first sign
- Mild ear pain or discomfort
- Ringing in the ears common

Nurse's order:
- Use OTC earwax kits to loosen and drain excess earwax
- Avoid using cotton swabs to clean the ear

## Ringing in the ears.

A continuous noise in the ear(s) that people describe as ringing, roaring, or buzzing—called tinnitus (TIN-uh-tus)—affects about 50 million Americans. It can happen after exposure to loud noise. If, for example, after enjoying a concert or attending an auto race you still hear a sound like the roar of the crowd when you get into your quiet car or back home, that's tinnitus. You're lucky when it goes away in an hour or so. If you are a big race fan and often go to the track, or attend loud concerts regularly, use earplugs to protect your hearing, just as people who operate jackhammers do. Many rock stars wear ear protection on stage, and many of the more senior rockers have serious hearing loss. Your ears may also "ring" if you take too much aspirin, which can happen to people taking high-dose aspirin therapy under the supervision of their HCP for treatment of a condition such as rheumatoid arthritis. The sound is most notice-able when you're in a quiet place, and only you can hear it. Drop the aspirin dose, and the noise will be gone in about a day.

### Hearing loss.

More than 28 million Americans have some degree of hearing loss. There are two types of hearing loss:

- Sensorineural, the term used for a problem with the structures behind the eardrum or the acoustic nerve that sends sound sig-nals to the brain.
- Conductive, the term used when sounds can't reach the eardrum and inner ear. The most common culprit? Earwax packed in the ear canal. However, certain infections and fluid in the ear can also cause conductive hearing loss.

## ❓ Frequently Asked Questions

Q. If I can't use a Q-tip, how can I clean my ears?
A. Actually, your ear is designed to clean itself quite nicely. If every-thing is normal, you shouldn't need to do much ear cleaning. If you do have wax buildup, see Self-Care (page 20).

Q. Is there a way to treat tinnitus?
A. If a work-up does not identify a treatable cause, tinnitus is now being managed with tiny devices similar to hearing aids that can be set at different frequencies to mask the tinnitus noise. If tinnitus does not go away after you've been exposed to loud noise at a race track or con-cert, call your HCP to get your hearing checked.

## TECHNICALLY SPEAKING . . .

The Eustachian tube connects the middle ear to the throat. It provides a path through which pressures can equalize, preventing pressure build-up behind the eardrum. When your ears "pop" in a plane or when you're driving into areas with higher elevation above sea level, that is pressure releasing through the Eustachian tube. If this tube gets blocked, trouble follows. What blocks it? Most commonly, swelling from allergies or a cold virus.

Unrelieved middle ear pressure can create a vacuum that draws fluid into the space, creating an ideal place for bacteria to grow. If pressure gets too high, the eardrum can rupture. Sometimes an HCP will make an opening in the eardrum to relieve pressure before it ruptures.

## NURSE'S WISDOM

- Don't automatically attribute ear pain to something wrong with your ear; remember that the actual source of the problem could be your teeth, sinuses, jaw, or tonsils.
- There is some debate about whether antibiotics should be prescribed for every earache with a bulging eardrum. In some cases, the pain is caused by a fluid collection and not an infection. Don't insist on a prescription if your HCP gives you an explanation as to why it's not warranted after an exam.
- Resist the urge to get a diagnosis over the phone and have a prescription called in. A painful ear deserves a look.
- When you apply heat to a sore ear, it can loosen the wax and cause it to run out of the ear. That's normal.
- Never flush your ear with cold water. It can stimulate a reflex that will make you very dizzy and even vomit.
- Roll a bottle of eardrops between your palms to warm the fluid to body temperature, just before it goes in your ear.
- Hydrogen peroxide isn't the best ear cleanser. When the oxygen fizzes away, it leaves water in the ear, which is what causes "swimmer's ear" in the first place. If you use hydrogen peroxide, follow up with a few drops of rubbing alcohol to dry the ear canal.

■ Check the label carefully and know the difference between eardrops and eyedrops; mixing them up is more common than you might think.

## SELF-CARE

For all simple ear pain, try applying heat with a warm washcloth or a heating pad set on low. Do not fall asleep on the heating pad! Take the OTC pain medicine you prefer—acetaminophen, aspirin, or ibuprofen. Never insert anything into the ear unless it is to put in eardrops.

### Ear infection (middle ear):
■ Use prescriptions as ordered. If antibiotic pills are prescribed, be sure to take every last one, even if you feel fine after a few days.
■ Sleep with your head propped up to help the middle ear drain.

### Ear infection (outer ear):
■ Keep your ears dry; shake your head to drain the water after a shower, or gently dry the ear using a hairdryer on low held about 18 inches away.
■ Make protective drops: combine equal amounts of rubbing alcohol and white vinegar, and put a few drops in each ear with a dropper after showering or swimming. You can also buy OTC drops for this purpose.
■ Limit the use of earplugs that block the ear and hold water in.
■ Treat any skin conditions that may contribute to the problem, such as eczema or psoriasis.

### Airplane ear:
■ Swallow frequently. Think about yawning, and you will. Both of these tricks often release the pressure most effectively. Chewing gum and sucking on hard candy also work.
■ If you're sensitive, don't sleep during takeoffs and landings,

when the pressure changes are greatest. You're less likely to swallow when you're asleep.

- If you have allergies or are congested, take a decongestant a few hours before takeoff to keep the Eustachian tube open.

### Earwax buildup:

- Mineral oil warmed to body temperature (no microwave) can soften earwax. Put a few drops in each ear twice a day.
- After softening the wax, try flushing it out by directing the warm water flowing from a showerhead into your ear.
- If these steps don't work, try an OTC earwax softener and gently flush the ear with warm water and an ear syringe. Use only a syringe designed for this purpose.

### Ringing in the ears:

- If you take aspirin every day as prescribed, check with your HCP about reducing the dose.
- Talk with your pharmacist (or check online) to see if any medicines you're taking could cause ringing in the ear.
- Minimize your exposure to loud noises and be sure to wear ear protection when mowing the lawn, riding the subway, or at loud recreational events.
- Avoid smoking cigarettes or drinking alcohol or caffeine—all can make the noise worse.
- If the noise makes it hard for you to sleep, play classical music or get a radio that also plays nature sounds to mask the noise.

## LISTEN UP!

Follow the old saying and never put anything in your ear canal smaller than your elbow.

# EYE IRRITATION AND VISION CHANGES

## NURSE'S NOTE

It's simple—you get two eyes, and that's it. So don't mess around when there's a problem. Eye symptoms need to be addressed promptly, whether it means calling your HCP or going to the ER. You should also have a personal or family ophthalmologist—an "eye MD." If you wear eyeglasses or contacts, it's fine to have your vision checked by an optometrist, but you should have a complete eye exam by an ophthalmologist early on—typically at the end of high school, and then as often as recommended based on any risk factors you may have for eye diseases such as glaucoma.

There is no condition for which rubbing your eyes helps, and in many cases, you can do harm by rubbing. I know it's virtually impossible not to rub your eyes since you may not even realize you're doing it. But think about it next time your eyes are bothering you.

## GET THEE TO THE ER

You don't necessarily have to call 911, but have someone give you a ride or go with you by mass transit if:

■ Something is in your eye and it doesn't come out with an eyewash, particularly if there's a visible speck on the eyeball.
■ You feel like there is something in your eye but can't see a speck. A scratch on the eye's surface (called a corneal abrasion) feels just like a grain of sand in the eye. It's common in contact lens wearers.
■ You have eye pain, and the area around the eye on your face is red, hot, and swollen.
■ You have a sudden loss of vision, have lost part of your visual

field (for example, you can see straight ahead, but nothing on the side), or you have the feeling that a curtain is being raised or lowered in your field of vision.

■ You're in pain, and your eye is sensitive to light, with or without blurred vision.

■ Your vision is impaired after a head injury.

■ You suddenly develop double vision.

## CALL YOUR HEALTH CARE PROVIDER

For many eye conditions, try a quick call to your ophthalmologist to see if you can meet him at the office rather than going to the ER. Conditions that can be handled with an initial phone call include:

■ A sty that blocks your vision.

■ A significant increase in the number of floaters in your eye.

■ Dry eye that doesn't respond to OTC eyedrops.

■ Problems related to contact lenses that don't involve an eye injury, such as a corneal abrasion.

■ An increase in eye irritation.

■ Your vision becomes blurred or changes in any other way.

■ If you have eyeball pain, not just irritation.

■ Any eye symptoms lasting longer than seven days.

## INSIDER INFO

■ If you have eye symptoms *not* caused by injury, call your ophthalmologist first. That office will have more equipment to perform a complete eye exam than the ER does. If you can, get an emergency appointment (and almost all offices hold slots open during the day if you really need to be seen). Otherwise, talk to the specialist on the phone and she'll let you know whether to meet her at the office, or if you should go to the ER instead. If you are having an eye problem, do not drive! However, if you have any of the conditions listed above, and you can't contact an ophthalmologist right away, don't wait, come in.

## COMMON CAUSES OF EYE IRRITATION

### Conjunctivitis (also called pinkeye).
This is an inflammation of the membrane that lines the eyelids and covers the eyeball. It can be caused by bacterial or viral infection, allergies, and other irritants. If the cause is an infection, it is *highly* contagious, so careful hygiene is essential. Be sure to wash your hands thoroughly if you have to touch your eyes.

How you feel:
- Eyes are irritated and bloodshot
- Vision seldom impaired

Other indicators:
- Drainage clear with irritation or allergy, or more thick and pus-like with infection
- Eyelids stuck together or crust on eyelashes when you wake up

Nurse's order:
- Apply warm compresses to clean eyes of crusts or drainage
- Avoid wearing contact lenses or eye makeup
- Call HCP if no improvement in 48 hours despite self-care

### Dry eye.
In this condition, eyes lack moisture. Dry eye is a common side effect of antihistamines and birth control pills. It can also occur if you work at a computer because you blink far fewer times per minute when you are focused on the screen than at other times. Ten million Americans have dry eye syndrome.

How you feel:
- Eyes are dry and irritated, and may burn
- Vision is not impaired

Nurse's order:

- Moisten eyes with OTC artificial tears
- Follow up with HCP if OTC artificial tears do not relieve symptoms

**Sty.**

This is a bump, like a pimple, on the eyelids or the edge of the lid caused by an infection at the base of an eyelash. They're very common and, like a pimple, usually come to a head, drain, and go away.

---

**? Frequently Asked Questions**

**Q.** *What are floaters?*

**A.** Floaters are stray cells or little bits of protein within the eye that float across your field of vision. Just about everybody has them, and you'll no doubt see more when you are thinking about it and looking for them. Mention it to your HCP the next time you visit, and if you see flashing lights or permanent marks in your vision, have it checked out promptly.

**Q.** *Sometimes my eye twitches. What does that mean?*

**A.** Eye twitches are muscle spasms of the tiny muscles around the eye, typically those around the outside corner. They can spasm when you are overtired or under stress. It's nothing to worry about unless it lasts continuously for more than a day. Then, touch base with your HCP.

**Q.** *I am getting older and need bifocals, I have astigmatism, or (fill in the blank). That means I can't wear contacts, right?*

**A.** Wrong! If you want contact lenses and haven't had an evaluation in a few years, check again. A number of technical advances now allow people with a variety of vision problems to wear contacts. My contacts fix my astigmatism and give me both magnification for reading and improved distance vision.

If the sty swells enough to impair your vision or doesn't improve despite self-care, contact your HCP.

## A NOTE ABOUT CONTACT LENSES

If you wear contact lenses every day, make sure you have a backup pair of eyeglasses! You never know when an injury, mild infection, or irritation can occur, meaning you need to put the contacts away for a few days. I can't tell you how many times I've told patients they needed to leave their contact lenses out for a few days, and they told me they had no eyeglasses. It never dawned on them that they might need them. Putting anything in your eye when there's a problem (other than medication, of course) can cause serious complications.

Wearing contact lenses means you must be responsible and keep your eyes healthy. As a lens wearer and nurse who's cared for my share of eye problems, my key rules are:

- Be meticulous about cleaning lenses if you don't wear disposable, single-use lenses.
- Never, ever touch your lenses or eyes until you have washed your hands thoroughly (or use one of the waterless hand sanitizers).
- Get an annual eye exam by an optometrist or ophthalmologist who has experience with contact lens wearers, knowing what special things to look for that are unique to contact lens wearers.
- Have that backup pair of eyeglasses.

If you wear contacts for cosmetic reasons, you may also want to wear glasses instead of contacts if you're just spending the day around home to give your eyes a break. If you're working at your computer, eyeglasses are a wise choice over contact lenses.

You may also want to look into daily disposable lenses. Since you put in a brand new pair every day, there's no cleaning required so the risk for infection is much lower than with traditional lenses. The clarity of vision is great.

## Did You Know?

Contact lenses can be permanently stained and ruined by medications that change the color of body fluids and by dyes used to examine the eye. The two most common drugs are Rifampin, an antibiotic used to treat tuberculosis or exposure to meningitis; and Pyridium (phenazopyridine), used to decrease pain from bladder spasms when you have a bladder infection.

Fluorescein eye stain, used to facilitate eye exams, will also dye contact lenses a yellow-orange color. Waterproof mascara can stain lenses the color of the mascara.

## NURSE'S WISDOM

- Many medical conditions affect your eyes. Some diseases with eye complications—such as diabetes—are well known. Others are less well known, such as dry eye associated with a skin condition called rosacea. Ask about potential for eye involvement with any new diagnosis and whenever you get a new prescription, particularly if you wear contact lenses or work at a computer all day.
- Medicines that list "dry mouth" as a side effect are also likely to dry your eyes.
- Antihistamines will dry your eyes as they dry all the fluids in your body.
- Many people can't keep their eyes open to put drops in. If you're one of those people, first make sure your eyelids are clean (thoroughly remove any eye makeup). Then, lie on your back and, with your eyes closed, squeeze the bottle to put the drop in the inside corner of your eye. When you open your eyes, the drop will flow in.
- To get the best concentration of medicine in the eye, immediately after the drop is in the eye, squeeze your eyelids tightly

together. Or squeeze the bridge of your nose near the inner corner of the eyes to block the tear duct that can drain the medicine.

- Do not touch the tip of any eyedrop bottle with your hands, and don't allow it to touch anything else because the tip is sterile. Take special care not to touch the tip to the eyelid or eyelashes. Put the cap back on immediately.

## SELF-CARE

### Conjunctivitis:

- Remember how contagious infectious conjunctivitis is, and wash your hands before and after you touch your eye(s). Don't rub your eye(s).
- Using a single, moistened cotton ball to wipe drainage from the eyelid and eyelashes. Sweep from the inside corner to the outside corner, using each cotton ball only once. Throw it in the trash immediately; don't let them pile up around the sink before you toss them.
- Apply cold or warm compresses to the eye(s) a few times each day (whichever makes you feel better), taking care to separate these washcloths from other laundry, and wash them in hot water.
- Do not wear eye contacts or eye makeup until the symptoms are completely gone for about 48 hours.
- Discard and replace any eye makeup that might have been contaminated.
- Never share eye makeup (under any circumstances), and don't share washcloths, towels, or handkerchiefs with someone who has conjunctivitis. Wash pillowcases in hot water and change them frequently. Also change the sheets once the infection is cleared up.
- If the inflammation is caused by an irritant, avoid exposure whenever possible.
- Don't go swimming while you're potentially contagious.

**Dry eye:**
- Use OTC artificial tears eyedrops.
- Stay away from irritants such as cigarette smoke, or air blowing in or on your face (such as from an air conditioning duct).
- If your allergy symptoms are limited to itchy, burning eyes, use antihistamine eyedrops instead of taking a pill that will affect your whole body.
- Drink plenty of fluids. Water is best.
- Take a break. If you work at a computer, plan times away from the screen when you might return telephone calls, do filing or take care of some other task that gets your eyes off the screen.

**Sty:**
- Apply warm, moist compresses to shrink the sty or bring it to a head so it will drain. Either will relieve discomfort. You can also apply a wet tea bag for relief.
- Don't rub the eye or squeeze the sty in an attempt to drain it.
- Avoid eye makeup or contact lenses until the condition is resolved.

## EYE IRRITATION REMEDIES

Self-treatment with eyedrops should only be for very minor conditions, or to wet contact lenses as directed by your optometrist. If your eyes are dry without an obvious cause, have your eyes checked. A number of medical conditions can cause dry eyes, and dry eyes can be a side effect of many medications. Untreated dry eyes can put you at risk for further eye irritation and injury.

In addition to the three types of eye medication drops, there are also artificial tears and rewetting drops that add moisture.

### Antihistamine.
Antazoline and pheniramine maleate are both antihistamine eyedrops. They reduce the itching and redness in the eyes caused by allergies. If your allergy symptoms are limited to your eyes, or if your

eyes bother you the most, you can use these medications and avoid the side effects that affect many parts of your body when you take antihistamine pills. They may burn at first when you put them in; that's normal when your eyes are irritated.

### Decongestant.

Just like decongestant pills, decongestant eyedrops, including naphazoline and oxymetazoline, shrink tiny blood vessels. The drops work on the white area of your eye (called the sclera) to reduce congestion, redness, and that bloodshot appearance.

### Astringent/Analgesic.

Zinc sulfate promotes tissue healing and shrinks tiny blood vessels, reducing congestion in the eye; these actions also reduce pain and discomfort from eye irritation. It reduces redness and bloodshot eyes, too.

### Eye lubricants.

These were once only available by prescription but are now available OTC for treatment of dry eye under the care and direction of your ophthalmologist. These are much thicker than other eyedrops and will make vision blurry for five to ten minutes after application. Ask your HCP if these drops are right for you. Do not use them as a substitute for an eye exam.

## ➕ When to Consider

- Use antihistamine drops for treatment of itchy eyes related to allergies.
- Use decongestant drops to decrease the appearance of bloodshot eyes.
- Use one of these four medications to treat the cause and to soothe irritated eyes
- Use artificial tears to moisten dry eyes.

## 🚫 Do Not Use

- Do not use eye medication if your eye irritation or redness is associated with pain, blurred vision, or other visual changes.
- Do not use eye medication while you are wearing contact lenses. (But remember you shouldn't be wearing contact lenses if your eyes are so irritated you need drops!)
- Do not mix prescription eyedrops with OTC eyedrops without consulting your ophthalmologist.

## LISTEN UP!

Granted, some people are lucky. But if you are not meticulous about washing your hands before you apply anything to your eyes, you *will* end up with an infection. Wash your hands, and don't touch the tip of eyedrops bottles to your eye, eyelid, skin on your face, or any surface that can contaminate it. Keep the cap visible, such as on a table, and replace the cap as soon as you've put the drops in your eyes. And, don't mess around. If your eyes aren't back to normal in a few days, see an ophthalmologist.

# TOOTHACHES AND MOUTH PAIN

## NURSE'S NOTE

As a true dental-phobe who can't sit in a dentist chair without my customized hypnosis tapes, I am close to breaking out in a sweat just writing this. If you feel the same way, you understand exactly what I mean. But that's no excuse to neglect your dental and oral care.

If you have dental problems, don't settle for a so-so dentist. Once you find a great dentist (by asking everyone you know and researching "best dentist" lists), you can then build your team with a root canal specialist and oral surgeon (if you've neglected your teeth, you'll probably need both). Once your dentist gets to know you, he or she can refer you to specialists who will take good care of you personally and do top-notch work in your mouth as well.

## GET THEE TO THE ER

Mouth problems rarely call for emergency care, yet many people go to the ER when they have a bad toothache. The problem is that ERs aren't equipped to do dental care. They'll just tell you to see a dentist in the morning. If you have a dental emergency, call your dentist first. He'll have the equipment to manage a variety of problems.

## CALL YOUR HEALTH CARE PROVIDER

- If your cold sore doesn't go away after a week or ten days.
- If you have a cold sore and eye pain or a change in vision. The infection may have spread to your eye.
- If you have sores in your mouth, a fever above 101 degrees, and/or chills.
- Call your dentist for any dental emergency or severe pain before going to the ER; the dentist is much better equipped to manage a dental condition.

## INSIDER INFO

There is a great deal of research showing a relationship between dental disease and illnesses such as heart disease, stroke, diabetes, and inflammation of the pancreas. In one comprehensive study, people with periodontal disease had a significantly higher incidence of heart disease, stroke, and premature death than those who had healthy mouths.

## COMMON TYPES OF DENTAL AND MOUTH PROBLEMS

### Toothache.

A toothache typically comes in three varieties:

1) A miserable constant ache caused by something as simple as that popcorn hull stuck between your teeth, or decay or an abscess beneath the tooth. An abscess can be extremely painful (to the point of interfering with sleep) because pus collects in a closed space in your gum or jaw. The resulting pressure causes intense pain since swelling cannot dispel the pressure here.

2) You see stars when you bite down or the dentist touches a cracked filling or cracked tooth. Cracked fillings are easy to replace. Cracks (also called fractures) in the tooth are not so simple. The tooth may have to come out if the fracture is vertical and goes into the root. If the fracture is horizontal, the tooth can be saved. Typically, you'll need a root canal, then the tooth is covered with a crown.

3) Sensitivity to cold can occur in normal teeth. It can also result from excessive tooth brushing, tooth decay, or receding or infected gum tissue. Products used to whiten your teeth can cause sensitivity as well.

### Tooth knocked out.

If a tooth is loose, call your dentist immediately. If an injury knocks out a tooth, find it, and call the dentist immediately. There is debate among experts whether it is best to place the tooth between the gum and jaw (as long as there is no chance you'll swallow it) to keep it moist with saliva, or to put it in a glass of milk. What's essential is that you don't let it dry out. Handle it as little as possible, and then only by the biting surface. Don't touch the root.

### Bad breath.

A number of factors can combine to cause bad breath. They include foods, such as onions and garlic; bacteria mixed with food particles (a.k.a. "morning breath"); smoking; dry mouth (saliva cleans the mouth and removes particles that cause odor); dental diseases and infections; and medical diseases such as respiratory infections, diabetes, and acid reflux from the stomach. You can cover your bad breath with mouthwash, but if a friend or loved one tells you your breath is bad, it's best to seek out the cause and treat that.

## Cold sore (also called a fever blister).

Cold sores are caused by a herpes simplex virus infection. And they are contagious. As one of my nursing instructors said, "If you have a cold sore, be sure to keep your mouth above your waist—or anyone else's," because herpes can be transmitted to other mucous membranes. Because cold sores are a viral infection, the first time you have an outbreak, you'll likely feel sick and have swollen glands. Most people don't remember this because it usually happens before age seven. Then the herpes virus will wait silently in your mouth until you have a fever from another illness, are under stress, or get a lot of sun exposure because you forgot to put sunblock on your lips. In some people, certain foods may trigger a cold sore—you'll learn which foods they are for you. Almost everyone has had a cold sore at least once by adulthood, and they know the telltale tingling or itching that occurs just before a sore appears. Cold sores are known for popping up at the most inopportune times—before an important job interview, before a big family get-together, even before your wedding! The common denominator? Stress.

How you feel:
- Itching or tingling sensation on lips or nearby skin
- Red swelling on the lips and nearby skin
- Swelling develops into painful red blisters

Nurse's order:
- Start treatment with OTC docosanol (Abreva) at the very first sign of an outbreak, even if you don't see a sore.
- Take HCP-prescribed antiviral medications

## Canker sore.

Unlike cold sores, canker sores are not contagious. Instead, they're caused by injury or irritation in the mouth—from spicy foods, from pizza that's too hot and burns the roof of your mouth, from a sharp edge on a tooth, from biting your tongue (particularly when your mouth is numb after dental work), or from food allergies or nutritional deficiencies.

How you feel:
- Sometimes painful sores in the mouth that are white, gray, or have a yellow crater in the center (Note that these are in the mouth, while cold sores are on the lips.)

## ? Frequently Asked Questions

Q. *What's the best toothbrush?*
A. That's like asking what's the best vacation spot! In this case, what's "best" for you is highly individualized depending on your age, the condition of your mouth and teeth, and your hand dexterity. Ask your dentist for a recommendation, and whether she thinks a manual or electric toothbrush is right for you. Harder bristles aren't necessarily better; they can injure delicate tissues.

Q. *Is my cold sore still contagious if I treat it with ointment?*
A. Yes! That's a critical point to remember. Abreva works to protect cells by creating a barrier to the virus at the cellular level. This action shortens healing time but does not mean you can't pass the virus on to others. Wash your hands before you apply the ointment and again after you've touched the area. Discard the tube of any medicine or lip moisturizer that touched the cold sore area, and have a new tube of docosanol on hand since you never know when you'll feel that telltale tingling. Never share lip moisturizers or balm, lipstick, or any medicines you use on your lips or mouth.

Nurse's order:
- OTC mouth ointments to treat pain and irritation

## TECHNICALLY SPEAKING ...

Bad breath after eating foods doesn't actually come from the mouth. Foods you eat are digested and absorbed into the bloodstream. When the blood reaches the lungs, the odor crosses into the lungs, where it is exhaled. Brushing, flossing, and gargling with mouthwash won't make much of a difference; you have to wait until the food leaves the body.

## NURSE'S WISDOM

- Gently used tea bags have tannic acid, which may shorten a cold sore outbreak if you apply the tea bag during the "tingle phase" before the full breakout; it may also soothe a canker sore.
- Avoid salty, spicy, or highly acidic food and drinks such as citrus fruits and coffee when you have any sores in your mouth.
- If you apply petroleum jelly to cover and protect a blister, use a cotton swab. Put the cotton swab in the jar to collect a glob of jelly, then apply the jelly to the blister *with the swab*. Never put the swab back into the jar as that will contaminate the whole jar and you'll have to toss it. Keep your fingers out of the jar for the same reason.
- Never, ever use lipstick "testers" in a store on your mouth.
- Keeping lips moist (with petroleum jelly or other moisturizers) and covered with sunblock can help reduce the number of cold sore outbreaks.

## SELF-CARE

### Toothache:
- If your teeth are sensitive—and you don't have a problem that requires a dental exam or you've been cleared by the dentist— use toothpaste designed for sensitive teeth. Think twice about tooth whitening, which increases sensitivity.

■ Don't abandon oral hygiene when you have a toothache or mouth sore. Brush gently in the affected area, or use an irrigator or mouthwash if the area is too sensitive to brush.

■ Try flossing in case a tiny piece of trapped food is causing the pain.

■ Apply a cold pack to your face or jaw over the toothache (or after major dental work if you're sore after the local anesthesia wears off).

■ Never apply heat to your face or jaw, unless it is specifically recommended by your dentist after an exam. Heat can increase swelling and pain.

■ Take the OTC pain reliever of your choice; do *not* put an aspirin right on the gum, which is an old wives' tale.

■ OTC remedies for toothache pain (numbing gel) can be effective. Use them *until* you can see your dentist, not *instead* of visiting your dentist.

■ Select soft foods of neutral temperature; chew on the side of the mouth that isn't sore.

## Bad breath:

■ Stay away from foods and drinks known to cause bad breath. These include garlic, onions, anchovies, hot peppers, salami and other spicy foods, and alcoholic beverages.

■ Brush and floss at least twice a day; if you have problems with dexterity and can't floss, use an irrigator instead.

■ Don't forget to brush your tongue.

■ Don't use any tobacco product. Stop smoking. Also, chewing tobacco not only causes bad breath, it can also cause mouth cancer.

■ Keep your mouth moist. Drink lots of water throughout the day.

## Cold sore:

■ Cold sores are contagious! Don't kiss people if you have a sore or feel that telltale tingling before a sore actually appears. Don't share towels, drinks, eating utensils, lip balm, or anything that may have touched your blister (or someone else's).

- Apply an ice cube to the sore (don't apply a reusable cold pack as you could contaminate it).
- Use OTC remedies to relieve cold sore symptoms. If you buy a product with an applicator, get the smallest size. You'll need to discard it after the outbreak.
- Once the outbreak is over, throw out your toothbrush and tube of toothpaste. If you get sores frequently, consider using the small tubes to avoid waste.
- Ask your HCP about a prescription for an antiviral cream you can apply to the sores (for example, Zovirax and Denavir).

**Canker sore:**
- Rinse your mouth with warm salt water (8 ounces to a teaspoon of salt). Don't swallow!
- Make a paste from baking soda and a few drops of water and apply it to the sore, or coat with a liquid antacid.

## MOUTH PAIN REMEDIES

Cold sores, canker sores, pizza burns—they all hurt, and make it difficult to eat and drink. OTC remedies for mouth problems either numb the painful area or, in one case, speed the healing of cold sores. Other products you'll find on the shelf can cover the sore with a coating you can "paint" on. Resist the urge to apply the symptom-relief medications more often than the label directs. Time is still going to be the best healer.

These remedies will not remove the blister; the mark is often the most troubling aspect of cold sores for many people. And, while nothing can cure the herpes virus, docosanol inhibits the virus's spread.

### Numbing.
Benzocaine, a local anesthetic, is available in many formulations—dental paste, lozenges, and liquid solution—for use in the mouth. Lidocaine is combined with camphor in a small patch that can be applied at the first sign of a cold sore to reduce pain and itching.

### Antiviral.

Docosanol (Abreva) is a cream that slows the spread of the herpes virus. It must be applied five times a day until the cold sore heals. While it does not contain an anesthetic, it speeds healing, and in some cases, can minimize blister formation if used early enough.

## ✚ When to Consider

- When you have a cold sore or feel the telltale tingling that precedes a breakout, use docosanol.
- When you have mouth pain caused by canker sores, dental appliances, temporary crowns, dentures or pizza burns, use a numbing medication in the formulation you prefer.

## 🚫 Do Not Use

- Do not use these OTC remedies for more than five days without checking in with your HCP or dentist.

## LISTEN UP!

If you get cold sores regularly, as soon as you feel that first tingle, start treatment to minimize the outbreak. Be particularly alert at times when you know you're likely to break out. Don't ignore a lump, bump, or sore in your mouth even if it doesn't hurt. And if you have a sore in your mouth that goes away on its own, comes back, and goes away again, don't assume everything is fine. Dental abscesses can behave that way. When the pressure in the abscess builds up, you'll get the bump on your gum; when it drains, the bumps goes away. Get it checked if a sore reappears after apparently healing.

# BODY ACHES AND PAINS

## BACK AND NECK PAIN

### NURSE'S NOTE

We nurses are intimately familiar with back pain because it's nearly impossible to lift and turn thousands of patients without feeling at least a twinge from time to time! But chances are that you've been down back roads, too. Four out of five of us will have significant low back pain at one time or another; half of us have it every year. The good news is that only about 5% of people who have back pain will need surgery. Since whole books are written on back pain, here I'll just cover the everyday, annoying, sometimes temporarily disabling pain. If you have a chronic condition, work with your HCP to map out a long-term plan of care, not a hit-or-miss plan for only when it acts up.

Keep in mind that there is no one solution for treating all types of back pain. If you use the Web as a resource in this area, be sure you know who owns the site you're visiting and what their perspective or bias is before you accept the information as expert advice.

## GET THEE TO THE ER

Dial 911 for back pain when:

- You've fallen and you can't get up.
- You have numbness below the waist and trouble walking.
- You have problems with your bladder or bowel; either losing control or not feeling when you need to go to the bathroom.
- You also have abdominal pain, and/or the skin below your waist is mottled or your feet are unusually cold and bluish.
- You have excruciating pain on one side in the soft part of the small of your back that shoots into your groin, with or without blood in your urine.
- You fell or were in an accident and also have significant neck pain.
- You have a stiff neck, headache, and fever, and the light hurts your eyes.

## CALL YOUR HEALTH CARE PROVIDER

- When you have pain with weakness below the knees. This should be true muscle weakness, not trouble moving your legs and feet because it hurts to do so.
- When you have pain that does not improve after 48 to 72 hours with appropriate self-care.
- When you have pain on one side in the soft part of the small of your back that may or may not shoot into your groin, foul-smelling urine, and a fever (you feel sick more than injured).
- When you have burning or aching pain in one side of the back, and you break out in a rash of itchy blisters over the area a few days after the pain starts.

## COMMON CAUSES OF BACK AND NECK PAIN

### Muscle strains.

Most commonly, back pain occurs when we lift something heavy, twist the wrong way, slip and fall, or otherwise strain the muscles.

If your back is strained to begin with, a simple sneeze can put your muscles into a painful spasm. If you're stiff when you wake up in the morning, your pain is most likely caused by a condition like arthritis. Wear and tear with age will cause gradual changes in the disks—the shock absorbers between the bones of the spine—that can cause pain. If a disk slides out of place, it's called a protruding, herniated, or slipped disk. It can press on nerves and cause leg pain, too. Disk problems are the most common reason for surgery, but not all disk problems require surgery.

How you feel:
- Pain intensity ranges from mild to severe
- Pain comes on gradually or suddenly
- If bad, pain hurts too much to move (may feel "locked up")
- Pain is felt anywhere from lower back up to neck
- Don't feel sick, just in pain

Nurse's order:
- Take OTC anti-inflammatory or prescription muscle relaxer

**Stiff neck.**
Like run-of-the-mill back pain, stiff necks are rarely serious unless you are also very sick. Waking up with a stiff neck is common if you have poor support from pillows while you sleep, or if you strain your neck because your workspace or home computer is not set up properly. The neck, shoulder, and back muscles are all connected, so stress that makes you subconsciously raise your shoulders can also stiffen your neck. (It can cause that tension headache, too! See page 4). Whiplash is the name given to a muscle spasm that typically occurs after your neck is quickly extended (your chin comes up) and then flexed (your chin goes down), as can happen in a car crash. There is currently debate about whether padded collars that don't allow neck movement are the best approach for treating whiplash.

How you feel:

- May not be able to move your head at all (especially when you wake up the morning after a fender bender)
- May be able to turn or move your head in only one direction, or only part way without feeling pain

Nurse's order:

- Moist heat: stand under a hot shower and gently turn your head as the hot water loosens the muscles
- Dry heat: electric heating pad or nonelectric heat source such as a ThermaCare Heat Wrap

**Kidney problems.**

Your kidneys sit on either side of your spine just below your rib cage. You can have significant kidney pain (in medical terms, called flank pain) from stones or an infection. A kidney stone stuck in the tube that connects the kidney to the bladder or in the tube leading from the bladder can make grown men cry. Often the urine will be bloody, and the pain seems to wrap around from the back to the groin.

A kidney infection, called pyelonephritis (PIE-low-neff-RIGHT-is), causes pain when the kidney swells. Kidney infections can come on quickly (in a matter of hours) with significant pain, fever, and foul-smelling urine; or gradually, particularly if a bladder infection has not been properly treated.

How you feel:

- Pain in back, side, groin, and/or genitals
- Pain is moderate to severe, and may come in waves
- Pain tends to come on suddenly
- Pain may make you sweaty and nauseated
- Pain hurts so much you can't lie still
- Pain is worsened by movement (going over a bump in the car)
- Blood in urine, visible or microscopic

Nurse's order:

- Drink plenty of fluids
- Take a prescription anti-inflammatory
- Get an opioid pain prescription
- Take a prescription antibiotic

## ? Frequently Asked Questions

Q. *What is sciatica (sigh-AT-uh-kuh)?*

A. It's an irritation, inflammation, or pinching of the sciatic nerve, which runs from your lower back through your buttock and down the back of your leg. Contrary to popular belief, pain in your leg does not automatically mean you have a slipped disk that needs surgery.

Q. *Should I see a chiropractor?*

A. That's often the question. I've worked with my chiropractor for more than 15 years; he has taken me from having spasms so bad that I almost crawled into his office to walking out the door about an hour later. I introduced my favorite orthopedic surgeon to him, and they refer patients back and forth regularly. But there is a real prejudice from many in the old guard medical community against chiropractors.

Would I go to my chiropractor to treat asthma or irritable bowel syndrome or irregular menstrual periods? No. My doctor of chiropractic is my back specialist. If I need a referral to a medical doctor, he picks up the phone. When I was searching for a new primary care provider, I ruled out a number of MDs because they refused to work with my chiropractor as part of my health team.

Q. *Which is better, babying that sore back or getting back in motion?*

A. A nursing research study showed that patients with acute low back pain who exercised for therapy missed fewer workdays than people who did no exercise therapy. If you're tempted to crawl in bed to wait out your back pain, don't! Exercise is best, but if you can't manage that, at least stay mobile and walk.

## SELF-CARE

If you have short-term low back pain, here's what an analysis of the research on treatments tells us.

It is *beneficial* to avoid bed rest and stay as active as you can. Take an OTC anti-inflammatory drug of your choice, or a prescription medicine from your HCP. It is *probably helpful* to use biofeedback to learn what muscle relaxation feels like and to get opinions from HCPs in different specialties who can provide different perspectives on your care (such as your family doctor and a chiropractor, or your regular nurse practitioner and an orthopedic specialist). Muscle relaxants are *helpful* but can cause significant drowsiness, limiting the usefulness of these drugs.

Treatment methods that are not yet proven to help, but *probably aren't harmful* to try include: acupuncture, pain medicine that does not relieve inflammation, massage, and ice or heat. (Timing of heat or cold therapy is critical. Using heat too early can cause swelling from the increased blood flow that may increase pain.) Bed rest is *harmful* because it weakens your muscles.

Back exercises may not be worth your time. Instead, overall fitness with a focus on abdominal muscle strengthening is far more important to provide support for your bad back.

If the treatment that works best for you isn't mentioned here, don't fret. It's important that you know what makes *you* feel better. Maybe next time, the researchers will call you!

## NURSE'S WISDOM

If you have chronic spasms, or if it doesn't take much to throw your back out:

- Bend both knees and hang on to a chair, desk, or countertop if you feel a sneeze coming on (and you're not sitting down). If you're lying down, pull your knees up to your chest for sneeze protection.

- Don't hold your breath because you hurt. Breathe slowly in through your nose, pucker up your lips, and breathe out slowly. Breath holding puts more pressure on your back muscles. The slow breathing can also help you relax.
- Lying flat on your back or flat on your stomach can be excruciating if your back is in spasm. Instead, curl up in the fetal position with a pillow between your knees. If you need to lie down for a scan or exam, here are the tricks: On your back, never leave your legs flat. If possible, put your feet flat on the table with your knees bent to take the pressure off the lower back. Otherwise, get your legs up on pillows. You can also consciously press the small of your back down and into the table, and release while you do your deep breathing. On your stomach, put a few towels underneath, right by your hipbones, to counteract the normal curve in your lower spine and relax the back.
- To relax the spasm, lie on your back on the floor or in bed with your knees pulled to your chest. Using a lot of pillows or something like a milk crate, gradually extend your legs so that you have a 90-degree angle at your hips and another 90-degree angle at your knees (like you're sitting in a chair while you lie on your back). I go to sleep in this position when I'm really in spasm.
- Repeated bouts of back muscle pain are usually less about your back and more about your abs. Weak abdominal muscles don't support your back as they should so you're more likely to strain muscles. Wear a strong support girdle to support both your abs and your back if you are going to be on your feet all day, or are doing things at work or around the house that could put your back at risk.
- Ask your HCP about getting custom orthotics for your shoes. A cast needs to be made of your foot (I've had them made by a physical therapist and a podiatrist). Two slim inserts will be designed—one for each foot's unique structure and posture. Then just slip them in your shoes. Orthotics correct even minor abnormalities in foot function or the length of your legs that can throw your back out over time, causing long-term

back pain. I got so much relief from my custom orthotics that I had a spare pair made just in case anything happens to my primary pair. I can't imagine going without them!

■ Freeze water in paper cups (about three-quarters full). When the pain hits, have someone massage the painful area with the ice. Your back partner holds the bottom of the cup, peels back the paper to expose the top of the ice, and rubs the ice where the pain is worst. Don't do it longer than seven to eight minutes each hour, and be sure to keep the ice moving to reduce the risk of frostbite.

■ Heat therapy (heating pad, Jacuzzi tub, hot pack) increases blood flow. For muscle strains and spasms, heat can help a lot. But be very cautious about using heat if you're not absolutely sure what's going on. It can make many conditions worse.

■ After the first 48 hours, try alternating heat and cold. Heat first to loosen muscles, then apply an ice chaser to reduce any swelling that the heat may cause.

■ If your back goes into spasm frequently, don't get into a hot bath or hot tub if you are alone. Think safety. What would you do if you couldn't climb out?

■ Even if you're pain free, never lie on your back and lift both legs off the floor 6 to 12 inches to strengthen your abs. That maneuver can easily tear small muscles in your lower back. Do abdominal curls, similar to sit-ups instead.

■ Consider a featherbed—the layer of bedding that goes on top of the mattress and under the fitted sheet—for added cushioning.

■ Some folks have had great success with a waterbed to reduce back pain, too. If you have found something that works for you, go for it!

If you spend a lot of time at a computer, set it up so you won't strain muscles:

■ The keyboard should be positioned so that you don't have to raise your arms to type. My wireless keyboard lets me put it on my lap, which is the best position for me. If you can't move the keyboard lower, sitting on a cushion may lift you to just the right angle.

- Don't hunch over the keyboard. Those knots will pop up between your shoulders. Instead, relax your shoulders, hold your head up, and keep your arms close to your sides.
- Keep your mouse as close to the keyboard as possible so you don't have to reach.
- Set your monitor at or a little below your natural eye level when seated in your workspace. If you have to lift your chin, you'll get a stiff neck.

If you have muscle or bone pain:

- Take it easy, but do not stay in bed or lie on the couch all day. Gradually work your way back to your normal activity level. Don't push it. Walk as much as you can.
- Use an anti-inflammatory OTC medicine of your choice. Do not take more than the recommended dose unless your HCP says otherwise.
- If you get relief from pain relieving rubs, gels, or creams, use the one you like best. Be aware that those containing capsaicin can irritate sensitive skin. Never apply heat when a rub is on the skin. Wash the rub off before applying any heat other than getting in a hot shower.
- Lying on your side or standing is less stressful for your back than sitting during the first two to three days of a pain episode. In the ER, I let folks stay in whatever position caused the least pain. Often, changing position hurts most.
- Apply ice for the first 24 to 48 hours; don't apply heat on your lower back until you have checked in with your HCP. Heat applied to a disk injury can cause swelling and make the pain and pressure on the nerves much worse. (I know. I did it and missed Christmas one year because the pain was so bad I couldn't walk.)

- Sleep on your side with a pillow between your legs. Never sleep on your stomach.
- For upper back pain between the shoulder blades, apply heat or stand under a hot shower, letting the hot water beat down on those painful knots.
- Relax. Chill. Be cool. Loosen up. Unwind. All that mental pressure usually goes directly to tighten your back muscles.
- Once the acute pain subsides, commit to a regular exercise program that will strengthen your abs, stretch your muscles to enhance flexibility, and improve your fitness. Minimize impact by walking, biking, or swimming.
- Work on maintaining a normal weight. Carrying extra pounds in front puts more pressure on the back.
- Learn how to protect your back. Bend at the knees to pick something up, never from the waist. Let those big muscles in your thighs do the work. Never twist at the waist while holding something heavy (like a bag of groceries or a shovel filled with snow); turn your whole body instead. Hold anything heavy close to your body for support. Use a luggage cart to wheel boxes around. *Don't hesitate to ask for help when you need it.*
- Get out of bed carefully in the morning, which is a high-risk time. First, pull your knees to your chest to stretch before you even try to get up. Then, roll over on your side and push yourself into a sitting position. Once sitting, you may want to bring your legs up to your chest again, hugging one knee at a time. Only then, push off with your hands to stand up.
- Choose your next car with care, particularly if you spend a lot of time behind the wheel. If you don't have a power seat that adjusts in 32 different directions, be sure to give your lower back some support. The easiest way is to roll up a towel and place it just below the small of your back near your tailbone. There are also fancier supports you can buy for car, office, and home.
- Stop and walk around at least 15 minutes for every 2 hours of driving.

- If you spend any amount of time on the phone for work, buy a headset. Not only is it far easier to multitask since your hands will be free, but not scrunching to hold the phone between your shoulder and ear will offer huge muscle benefits.
- Finally, if you want to reduce the number of back pain episodes, the high heels have to go. I've been a fashion "don't" for as long as I can remember. Sigh.

## LISTEN UP!

If you have a bad back, it can have a big impact on your life. There's no question that it can be debilitating. But in addition to the tips and self-care here, consider how you think and talk about your situation. If you say you "*Suffer from* back pain," you will! Try saying, "I'm *living with [coping with]* back pain" instead. See the difference? Instead of suffering as a victim, you are taking control to go on living your life despite the pain. Make back pain just one part of who you are; don't let it define you.

## INSIDER INFO

In the past year, the market has been flooded by various pain-relieving patches designed primarily to treat muscle pain. It is critical that you understand the difference among these products you can apply to your skin.

## PRODUCTS THAT GENERATE HEAT

Heat therapy dilates blood vessels which can reduce stiffness and reduce pain.

**ThermaCare Heat Wraps** are layers of clothlike material containing small discs that generate heat when they are exposed to the air. The temperature cannot go higher than 104 degrees, so you can't get burned. The pads provide heat for at least eight hours, so if you have a knot in your back, for example, you can put one on before you go to bed and get relief by morning. The wraps have adhesive and are applied directly to the skin.

**Cura-Heat and Bodi Heat** are also air-activated heat packs, but used differently than ThermaCare. These are applied to clothing over the area, rather than directly on the skin. They can get as hot as 127 degrees, and are not recommended for use while sleeping. The heat lasts as long as 12 hours.

## PRODUCTS THAT APPLY MEDICINE

These are patches containing common OTC medicines you can also purchase in tubes and apply as an ointment to the skin. The patches offer a no-muss, no-fuss way to apply the medicine of your choice. These ingredients are all considered to be counterirritants; they cause irritation or mild inflammation of the skin to distract the pain sensation from muscles or joints. Whether you are applying these medications by ointment, cream or patch, never apply heat over the same area of skin. You could more easily burn yourself.

**Icy Hot Patch** contains methyl salicylate and menthol. **Mentholatum Pain Relieving Patch** contains menthol. **Absorbine Jr. Patch** contains menthol, camphor, and eucalyptus, and **Therapatch** contains capsaicin.

# BONE, MUSCLE, AND JOINT PAIN

## NURSE'S NOTE

Problems with your bones, muscles, and joints are particularly troubling because the associated pain can make it hard to move around. But if you move less, you often hurt more, lose muscle mass, and become weaker, which can establish a vicious cycle.

I was diagnosed with fibromyalgia in 1991, and I actually don't remember what it's like to be pain free. Don't have a pity party for me, however. We all have challenges, and I certainly have not let my chronic problem stop me. Slow me down sometimes, yes, but stop me? No way. If you have a chronic condition such as arthritis or fibromyalgia, you've got to buck up and work through the pain because if you don't, you'll lose your flexibility and mobility for sure. A friend who has limited mobility from polio told me it's simply mind over matter—if you don't mind, it won't matter.

## CALL YOUR HEALTH CARE PROVIDER

- If you have a rash and fever with joint pain
- If you experience significant or new pain and swelling that does not go away or lessen with self-care.
- If you get sudden back pain and already know you have osteoporosis.
- If signs of carpal tunnel syndrome do not go away with self-care for a week or two.

## COMMON CAUSES OF BONE, MUSCLE, AND JOINT PAIN

### Osteoporosis.

With osteoporosis, bones lose thickness, become brittle, and are less able to support weight. Most commonly, the spine, hips, and wrists are hit hardest, and this is where broken bones are most likely to occur. While more women than men get osteoporosis, men are not immune. A lifetime of adequate dietary calcium along with vitamin D and weight-bearing exercises will help build and maintain strong bones.

How you feel:
- Bone pain in spine, hips, and wrists
- Pain with bone injuries

Other indicators:
- Bones can break easily
- Pain is not related to a specific time of day
- You experience no swelling
- You are over age 65

Nurse's order:
- Adequate calcium (1000-1300 mg/day) and vitamin D (400-800 IU/day )intake
- Limit smoking and alcohol use
- Take prescription meds to increase bone density if indicated

## Fibromylagia (FM).

This is a complex syndrome characterized by poor quality, non-restorative sleep, which leads to chronic muscle and joint pain and fatigue. The American College of Rheumatology has specific criteria for diagnosis, based on identification of "tender points" on both sides of the body above and below the waist. People with fibromyalgia may also have irritable bowel syndrome.

How you feel:
- Chronic muscle pain and fatigue
- Muscle pain in upper back, shoulders, and hips
- Poor sleep quality
- Morning stiffness
- Generalized warmth during flare

Other indicators:
- May be triggered by major injury or infection
- You are age 20 to 50

Nurse's order:
- Take OTC pain killers
- Prescription medicine to enhance sleep
- Prescription antidepressants can aid sleep and relieve pain

## Muscle cramp.

Sometimes called a "charley horse," this cramp occurs when the muscle contracts strongly, typically the large muscle of the calf. Pain is sudden and severe. The muscle is rock hard. Cramps can happen with overuse or dehydration. The muscle will reach the fatigue point within 60 to 90 seconds and the spasm will then stop. Stretching before exercise can reduce cramping; massage can break a cramp.

## Arthritis.

There are literally about a hundred types of arthritis, but I'll define the two most common: osteoarthritis and rheumatoid arthritis. You can think of osteoarthritis as a "wear and tear" condition. Over the years, the cartilage at the end of bones that come together in joints wears away. (Cartilage reduces friction and helps the bones slide past each other when you bend a joint such as your knee or those in your fingers.) When cartilage wears away, one bone can scrape against another, causing pain. Osteoarthritis can be a normal part of aging, or it can occur in a single joint that has been injured. Cartilage can also be worn away when subjected to stress—for example, research shows that arthritis in both knees is more common in overweight people of any age with more women affected than men. On the other hand, rheumatoid arthritis is an inflammatory disease in which the immune system attacks normal tissues; you may feel sick and have a low fever and lose weight when it flares up. Osteoarthritis only affects joints; rheumatoid arthritis can affect other parts of the body as well.

### *Osteoarthritis*
How you feel:
- Wear and tear on your body
- Morning stiffness
- Pain in your fingers, knees, hips, and back/spine area
- Chronic pain

Other indicators:

- You are age 45+
- There is no swelling
- There is no injury

Nurse's order:

- Take an OTC pain medicine of choice

### Rheumatoid arthritis

How you feel:

- Inflammation of hands, wrists, or feet (often warm to touch)
- Morning stiffness
- Chronic pain

Other indicators:

- There is no injury
- You are between the ages of 20 and 50
- There is swelling, redness, or warmth

Nurse's order:

- Take an OTC anti-inflammatory or other medicines as directed by your HCP

### Bursitis.

Bursae are fluid-filled sacs that cushion bones, tendons, and ligaments. A bursa helps a joint move smoothly in all directions. The sac can become inflamed after injury or overuse.

How you feel:

- Pain in one place with movement
- Short-term pain

Other indicators:

- No swelling or feelings of heat
- History of injury or overuse

Nurse's order:
- Take an anti-inflammatory, prescription or OTC

## Carpal tunnel syndrome.

This occurs when a nerve that travels through the wrist is compressed, often from overuse or holding your hands and wrists in the same position while doing the same activity over and over such as typing at a keyboard. Pain and numbness begins in the fingers (except the pinkie) and can be bad enough to wake you from sleep. Hand strength will also weaken over time.

How you feel:
- Numbness, weakness, pain in fingers
- Pain with repetitive motion of hand

Other indicators:
- No swelling or warmth
- Pinkie not affected.

Nurse's order:
- Take an OTC painkiller or anti-inflammatory drug

## Tendinitis.

Tendons connect muscles to bones. Injury or overuse can cause inflammation, swelling, and pain. Symptoms and treatment are very similar to bursitis.

How you feel:
- Pain in one place with movement
- Short-term episodes of pain

Other indicators:
- Often affects shoulder or elbow
- No swelling or warmth to touch
- History of injury or overuse

**Frequently Asked Questions**

Q. *Can my PCP give me an injection for joint pain?*
A. Bursitis is best treated with a single injection of corticosteroid if self-care does not relieve pain. A corticosteroid is a long-lasting, high-strength anti-inflammatory drug. Pain will increase significantly in the first 24 hours (so plan accordingly if you're getting an injection), but then usually quickly decreases.

Q. *Does carpal tunnel syndrome always need surgery?*
A. No. Changing the motions of the hands and positions of the wrists, sometimes with splints, can provide symptom relief without surgery.

Nurse's order:

- Take an anti-inflammatory, OTC or prescription

## NURSE'S WISDOM

- Women should discuss with their HCP ways to keep bones strong while they are in their 30s and 40s; a bone density test will pick up early stages of osteoporosis before X-ray evidence.
- Morning stiffness often responds to heat such as hot shower to loosen muscles and joints. Afterward, a routine of gentle stretching or yoga can help you get going.
- Do not apply heat to a joint that is swollen, red, or already warm to touch; use ice instead.
- A featherbed (or equivalent, if you have allergies) can provide cushioning and provide for more comfortable sleep.
- Non-weight–bearing exercises that emphasize balance and flexibility such as Pilates, t'ai chi, and yoga can be of great benefit, except for osteoporosis, in which weight-bearing exercise is needed to strengthen bones.

- If your hands are affected, look for household items that will make tasks easier such as large-handled kitchen utensils, an electric can opener instead of a manual one, large-barrel pens, and the like.
- If you think you have fibromyalgia, find a specialist who is experienced in working with people with FM and is up to date on treatment options. If you're feeling miserable and your HCP brushes you off because no "tests" are abnormal, find another HCP. Be careful about searching the Web for information about FM; not all the information is reliable or science based. (See Web Resources for an index to sites with reliable information.)

## SELF-CARE

### Osteoporosis:
- Maintain adequate intake of dietary calcium; look for calcium-fortified foods.
- Keep bones strong by doing weight-bearing exercises. Balance and stability are critical to preventing falls.
- If underweight, gain weight for balance and stability.
- Stop smoking and avoid drinking alcohol, which make bones more brittle.

### Fibromyalgia:
- Get enough sleep—this is the key to managing symptoms. The number of hours needed is different for each person with FM. If you're affected, you'll learn the amount of sleep you'll need to keep your symptoms at baseline.
- Stay active, but pace your activities. For example, I refuse to stay home because traveling to speak at seminars flares my FM; to me, the added pain is worth it because of the rewards I get from meeting and teaching colleagues all over the country. Getting up early to teach or be on a morning TV program is bad for FM, too. I've learned I need to build in at least one

"off day" after a trip or a day I have to get up early so my body can recover and I can get extra sleep. You need to find the balance that works for you.

■ Treat pain symptoms with the OTC pain reliever of your choice. There is no evidence of inflammation with fibromyalgia, so an anti-inflammatory medicines (such as ibuprofen, naproxen or ketoprofen) are not required, but they may work for you. I take aspirin daily to manage my pain.

## Arthritis:

■ Pain-relief creams and ointments applied to joints can decrease symptoms with minimal side effects. Take an OTC pain reliever as needed. As in fibromyalgia, osteoarthritis is not characterized by inflammation, but rheumatoid arthritis is. Thus, an OTC anti-inflammatory will not treat the cause of the pain in osteoarthritis, but it will if you have rheumatoid arthritis.

■ Maintain a healthy weight to minimize stress on hips and knees.

## Bursitis and tendinitis:

■ Rest the painful joint.

■ Take an OTC anti-inflammatory pain medicine of choice.

■ Apply a cold pack to the painful area; a typical schedule for an acute episode is 20 minutes of cold therapy every 2 hours during the day.

## Carpal tunnel syndrome:

■ Ice down wrist(s) after activities that increase pain, such as typing or other repetitive hand motions.

■ Take an OTC anti-inflammatory pain medicine of choice.

■ Switch activities as often as possible to change hand position (for example, separate periods of typing with other tasks such as making telephone calls).

■ Do regular stretching and flexibility exercises for hands and fingers. (See Web Resources.)

## LISTEN UP!

The good news is that some bone, muscles, and joint conditions—osteoporosis and carpal tunnel syndrome in particular—can be prevented if you're aware of the risk factors. Don't ignore early warning signs; the sooner you rest an overuse or inflammation condition such as carpal tunnel syndrome, tendinitis, and bursitis, the better your chances of a quick recovery.

## CHEST PAIN

## NURSE'S NOTE

The chest is a pretty complicated place because so many vital structures are located there. Typically, there are six sources of chest pain: heart problems, lung problems, trouble with swallowing, and pulled or strained muscles or rib injuries.

The bottom line is that if you are at all concerned that you may be having a heart attack, or your chest pain is making it hard for you to breathe, don't mess around. Call for an ambulance right away.

## GET THEE TO THE ER

A heart attack is an emergency. Call 911 if you have one or more of these heart warning signs:

- Pain in the middle of the chest and not in one small place you could point to with your fingers.
- A squeezing sensation in the chest.
- A feeling that there is a great weight on the chest, or a sense of pressure.
- Pain that moves from the chest into the shoulders or jaw.

- Pain, squeezing, or pressure during or immediately after physical exertion.
- Pain, squeezing, or pressure that awakens you from sleep.
- Pain, squeezing, or pressure plus dizziness, nausea, or trouble catching your breath.

Also call 911 if you:

- Have known angina that changes in that it lasts longer, doesn't go away with your prescribed nitroglycerin, or feels like a different type of pain.
- Have chest pain of any type and trouble breathing (particularly if you have recently had surgery or took a lengthy airplane or car trip).
- Have something caught in your throat, you can't swallow your own saliva, and/or your breathing is affected in some way such as you are experiencing repeated coughing, shortness of breath, or squeaking sounds when you breathe.
- Have chest pain and it is getting worse. You're not sure what's going on, but your instinct tells you it is something really bad.
- Feel palpitations and are lightheaded, like you're going to pass out.

## CALL YOUR HEALTH CARE PROVIDER

- If you have chest pain with a deep breath and cough, and generally feel sick.
- If your chest pain comes more than once a week after a meal, is more burning than painful, and you have a sour taste in the back of your mouth.
- If your discomfort is worse when you bend over from the waist or lie down.
- If you get heartburn after starting a new medication.
- If you have burning or aching pain on one side of the chest,

and you break out in a rash of itchy blisters over the painful area a few days after the pain starts.

## INSIDER INFO

Unless you go to the ER with chest pain that is obviously *not* heart related (for example, a bruised rib because you slipped in the bathtub), a heart attack will be assumed until proven otherwise. You'll get the EKG, heart monitor and the work-up for safety's sake. Don't be nervous about this.

If you think you may be having a heart attack, get to the ER ASAP by ambulance. It can be very difficult, even in the ER, to determine if pain is due to swallowing problems or poor blood flow to the heart, so don't try to diagnose yourself. I've taken care of far too many people who treated their heart attacks with antacids and waited 12 hours before coming to the ER. Delay can limit treatment options. For example, clot-buster drugs that relieve blockages in the blood vessels can only be used during a short window of time. If the blockage can be treated quickly enough with drugs or with a procedure such as angioplasty, heart cells can be saved.

It is becoming more common for people with chest pain who don't have an absolutely clear diagnosis to be kept for observation for about 23 hours so that their heart rhythm can be watched, and EKGs and other tests can be repeated to see if there are any changes from when they first came in. Don't stay away because of this potential; I just want you to know what to expect. That period of observation doesn't mean they're not telling you everything; it's just a precaution.

## COMMON CAUSES OF CHEST PAIN

### Heart pain.
Heart pain can occur suddenly, particularly during a heart attack. Or it may be something you have from time to time and after a medical work-up, you may be diagnosed with angina. People with sta-

ble angina who have had their heart checked out can usually go about their normal activities. If you have a prescription for nitroglycerin, be sure and keep it up to date and handy. If the pain (or the sensation you usually feel) occurs, takes it easy, sit or lie down, and rest. Take your nitroglycerin as directed and follow any other recommendations from your HCP.

How you feel:

- Pain in the chest area, or a sensation of continuous squeezing or pressure in the chest
- May be nauseated or even vomit
- Pain doesn't change when you move or change positions, you breathe in, or someone presses on the area that hurts most

Other indicators:

- Pain often comes on after physical activity or high anxiety or stress, or it can wake you from sleep

## Lung problems.

The lungs themselves are not particularly sensitive to pain, but tissues covering them are, and they will not be timid about letting you know when there's a problem. The most common chest pain from lung disease occurs when people have irritation or inflammation of the sensitive membrane covering the lungs, called the pleura (PLOORE-uh). That's where the name pleurisy (PLOORE-uh-see) comes from. If you have an infection such as influenza (see page 94) or pneumonia (see page 95), the pleura can become inflamed. You'll feel a sharp, stabbing pain in one place when you breathe in as the lungs expand and stretch the pleura. Most people learn very quickly just how small their breaths need to be to avoid triggering that pain.

How you feel:

- Sharp, stabbing pain in the chest only when you take in a breath or cough
- Pain is located in one place that you can point to with your finger

- Pain gets better if you breathe faster and with shallow breaths
- Pain gets worse if you breathe deeply, cough, or sneeze
- Pain doesn't change if you change positions or press on the area of most pain
- Sick from an infection

Other indicators:
- Pain often happens when you have a respiratory infection
- May or may not have fever

## Swallowing problems.

Swallowing problems can cause chest pain because the muscular tube that connects your mouth with your stomach—the esophagus (e-SOFF-a-gus)—runs through your chest behind your heart. Problems typically fall into two categories: something is stuck in the esophagus or acid from the stomach backwashes up into the esophagus.

### *Something stuck in esophagus*

How you feel:
- Pain comes suddenly while you're eating
- Pain or pressure occurs in the middle of your chest
- Unable to swallow your own saliva

Nurse's order:
- Visit the ER, where we call this an "across the room diagnosis" and ring up the specialist while you're still signing in

### *Reflux*

When you eat, your stomach produces more acid to digest the food. When the food fills the stomach and puts more pressure on the opening back to the esophagus, the acid may flow backward from the stomach into the esophagus and cause pain. The technical term for this is reflux.

If you've had four slices of a meat lover's deluxe pizza with

extra garlic after eating nachos with spicy jalapeño salsa and
drinking two beers, you may bring on a rousing case of heartburn.
That's to be expected, unless you have a cast-iron stomach. A
heartburn remedy and time will help you feel better. But if you are
having discomfort regularly and are taking a lot of OTC medicines
to treat yourself, you need to see your HCP as you may be experiencing reflux. What's "a lot?" If you're taking these remedies
every day or a few days each week or if you have to make sure you
always have them with you because your symptoms are so frequent, then that's a lot. If you have a cough associated with reflux
pain, see page 102.

How you feel:
- Burning sensation or pain in chest
- Burning sensation or pain that gets worse when lying down or
  after a meal
- Burning sensation or pain that is not affected by movement or
  breathing
- Burning in throat, or an acid or sour taste in throat and mouth
  especially after a burp

Other indicators:
- Discomfort worsens when you recline in an easy chair or lie
  down after eating

Nurse's order:
- Take OTC antacids for occasional symptoms
- Contact your HCP if your symptoms require an OTC stomach
  remedy for more than two weeks

## TECHNICALLY SPEAKING . . .

Acid backwash now has a fancy name, gastroesophageal (GAS-
troh-ess-OFF-uh-gee-ul) reflux disease or GERD. The special valve
between the esophagus and the stomach is called a sphincter. It is

supposed to stay closed except when you're eating; then it opens to allow food or drink to enter the stomach. If it doesn't stay closed, or it closes improperly, the normally acidic fluid that's in the stomach can go backward into the esophagus. The tissue that lines the esophagus wasn't designed to withstand the acidic fluid the way the stomach lining is, so the acid burns and irritates the esophagus. Since the pain is close to the heart, the original name, heartburn, was coined. Most people will have heartburn at one time or another. It becomes GERD when it happens frequently and when there is a firm diagnosis from your HCP.

### Broken rib bone or pulled muscles.

Ribs form the cage that protects the vital organs of the chest. They stand up pretty well to wear and tear, but sometimes do break. Breaks are most common in older people whose bones are more brittle, and in people who have experienced a sudden impact, such as from a fall or auto accident. You can also get bruised ribs.

Broken or bruised ribs don't appear out of thin air. You may forget slipping and falling in the bathtub at bedtime until you have pain the following morning, but think hard, and you should remember some sort of injury.

There are also many muscles between the ribs and around the rib cage. These muscles can get pulled or can go into spasm. When the muscles between the ribs go into spasm, it can be very scary because it can be difficult to breathe.

How you feel:
- Constant pain or ache in chest or rib area
- Pain felt after a fall or other injury
- Pain that gets worse with movement, when you breathe in, and when someone presses on the spot that hurts
- Discomfort that does not change with a change in body position
- Usually not sick

## ❓ Frequently Asked Questions

Q. *My son has something called costochondritis (COST-oh-con-DRY-tus). What is that?*

A. This is an inflammation of or injury to the area where the ribs are connected to the breastbone (called the sternum). Weightlifters often get it, as do people who participate in activities in which the arms are pulled backward, such as rowing. A key aspect of costochondritis is worsening pain when pressure is applied where it hurts, alongside the sternum. The condition is painful, but not dangerous, and is treated with anti-inflammatory medicines and applying heat and/or cold.

Other indicators:

- You can point to the spot that hurts with one finger
- Without realizing it, people with muscles and bone chest pain will breathe faster and take more shallow breaths to limit movement of the injured area

Nurse's order:

- Take OTC pain relievers
- Take OTC anti-inflammatory medication
- Apply heat or cold to relieve pain

## TECHNICALLY SPEAKING . . .

Sharp, stabbing lung pain can occur if the lung is partially collapsed. This can happen if you're in an accident of some sort, particularly if you have broken ribs that can puncture your lung. However, about 8,000 to 9,000 people—typically, healthy, young men, but it can happen to anyone—will experience a small tear in the lung for no apparent reason. If you suddenly feel a stabbing pain with a deep breath and shortness of breath but no symptoms of illness, it's worth a call to your HCP or visit to the ER or urgent care center for a chest X-ray. For more info, visit pneumothorax.org, a great site designed by a young man who's been through this himself.

## NURSE'S WISDOM

- If you have angina, keep the nitroglycerin close at hand. It doesn't do you any good if you're at the mall when you feel pain and your nitro is in the medicine cabinet at home. Many people keep a small bottle with a few tablets in their purse or pocket. You may want to keep one bottle in the car, so it will be handy. If you golf, for example, keep a bottle in your bag in case you get angina on the fifth hole well away from the clubhouse. Nitroglycerin pills have a very short shelf life and need to be replaced often. If you rely on nitroglycerin from time to time (but not often enough to need regular refills), you may want to establish a schedule, such as getting a new prescription when you turn the clocks ahead or back every year. Last year's nitroglycerin pills are pretty useless.
- Antacids coat your stomach and neutralize acid. That's a good thing. However, then can also block the absorption of many medications. To be safe, don't take pills with an antacid chaser. If you have questions about specific medicines, check with your HCP or pharmacist.

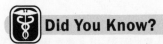 **Did You Know?**

A nursing research study of 183 people (ages 19 to 65+) was conducted to find out whether ER response time was the same for men and women who came in with heart attack symptoms. The results: 82% of men were brought into the ER treatment area within 15 minutes of talking to the intake nurse, while only 58% of women were. If you're a woman (or with a woman) having symptoms of a heart attack, you may need to be more assertive about being seen, since women have more subtle symptoms and because bias may exist.

■ Eating a few stalks of celery can help quench heartburn by absorbing acid.

## SELF-CARE

### Heart pain—Angina:
■ Relax. Stress increases the adrenalin in your body, and adrenalin makes your heart work harder. If your heart works harder, it needs more oxygen, which is a recipe for trouble.
■ Don't smoke. Nicotine produces more adrenalin and smoking damages your arteries.
■ Keep active. If you're a little nervous about exercising at first, ask your HCP about a cardiac rehab program in which your heart will be monitored so you'll learn your limits while having a specially trained nurse nearby. Walking is a terrific way to stay in shape.
■ Ask your HCP about taking a low-dose aspirin every day.

### Lung problems:
■ Breathe through your nose, and your body's natural filtering system will make it less likely that you'll be surprised by a cough. That reflex deep breath before the cough can be excruciating.
■ Take OTC anti-inflammatory drugs such as aspirin, or ibuprofen, naproxen, or ketoprofen.
■ Apply a pain relief rub or patch (see pp. 49–50)
■ Take it easy, and if the pain doesn't go away in a few days, see your HCP.

### Heartburn:
■ If you have heartburn after eating or drinking, you can take an OTC antacid that will neutralize the acid or an acid blocker that will reduce the amount of acid your stomach produces. Check with your HCP or pharmacist before making your choice; some of the acid reducers work more effectively if you take them before that "high-risk" food you just *have* to eat.

Learn the differences between the various stomach remedies available and which is right for you.

- If you need to treat your heartburn more than once a week, or after eating a variety of foods (not just that spicy meatball), have it checked out.
- Try eating smaller meals more frequently rather than one or two big meals a day.
- Wait a few hours after eating before you lie down or lean back in the easy chair.
- Avoid drinking coffee, carbonated drinks, or alcohol, and try to limit eating chocolate, tomatoes or tomato sauces, spicy foods, fatty or fried foods, peppermint or spearmint, or foods flavored with these mints. These goodies will either relax the valve (sphincter) that keeps acid in the stomach or they'll sit in your stomach for a long time, creating pressure likely to push acid upward. Consume them together, and a relaxed sphincter plus high stomach pressure means double trouble.
- Don't smoke.
- Unwind. Stress increases heartburn.

### Rib pain:
- Take OTC anti-inflammatory drugs.
- Initially apply ice to a muscle strain, spasm, or rib injury to reduce swelling and pain. If you use heat too soon, you'll increase blood flow, which increases swelling and pain. After about 48 to 72 hours, switch from cold to heat to speed muscle healing.
- After the cold phase, you can also try a pain relieving rub; do *not* use a rub and external heat at the same time because you could burn yourself.

## LISTEN UP!

Chest pain can be scary, especially if you know someone who has been hospitalized for a heart attack or bypass surgery or you have a family history of heart attacks. If you have any concerns about your heart, call 911. Otherwise, monitor your symptoms and contact your HCP if the symptoms don't go away in a day or two or if they're getting worse instead of better.

If you're having chest pain that requires an ER visit, don't drive yourself to the hospital or have someone else take you in a car. Call an ambulance. An ambulance will have the equipment on hand so you can have oxygen right away, and the crew can provide any additional care you may need on the way.

## WEAKNESS AND DIZZINESS

### NURSE'S NOTE

When a nurse asks "What's bothering you the most?" the answer "I feel weak all over and dizzy" often makes a diagnosis more difficult. Why? Because that description isn't specific enough. You might feel weak and dizzy for a simple reason: you skipped breakfast and so your blood sugar dropped. Or you might feel weak and dizzy because of something much more serious, such as a head injury. And of course, there's everything in between. Weakness and dizziness can even be the only symptom of anemia.

Telling your HCP you are weak and dizzy is really the equivalent of saying, "I don't feel good." Use this section to try to narrow down what you're really feeling. Then your HCP can be much more helpful, limiting the wild goose chase that can go with tracking down such generalized symptoms.

### GET THEE TO THE ER

You've earned a ride to the ER if:

- By weak and dizzy, you mean you remember feeling lightheaded and unsteady on your feet, then found yourself on the floor, but don't exactly remember how you got there (in other words, you passed out and fell down).

■ The weakness and dizziness came on suddenly and, at the same time, you have slurred speech, numbness, tingling, loss of movement or feeling on one side of your body, or abrupt changes in your vision, or a combination of any these symptoms.

■ The weakness and dizziness came on suddenly with another symptom, such as chest pain, a racing pulse, or an excruciating headache.

■ You're weak and dizzy after a head injury.

## CALL YOUR HEALTH CARE PROVIDER

■ If you think you're dehydrated.

■ If you develop vertigo (defined later in this section) and never had the sensation before.

■ If you get vertigo when you move your head too fast.

■ If you develop vertigo and a change of hearing at the same time.

■ If you are weak and dizzy days or weeks after a head injury.

■ If you have a change in hearing on one side.

■ If lightheadedness, vertigo, or dizziness comes on after starting a new medication.

■ If you have repeated spells of lightheadedness over a few days.

■ If weakness is related to a change in muscle strength or your ability to do certain tasks.

## COMMON TYPES OF WEAKNESS

There are two types of "weak," but they don't have any fancy names. Weak can mean that you feel washed out, fatigued, exhausted, have no energy, and that you would like to sleep for a week. (You know, how many of us feel on a daily basis.) The other weak is when you actually lose strength or are not able to use your muscles properly. Most of the time, it's the former.

Instead of only saying you're weak, describe how you feel—for example, "I am so weak that I can barely make it up the stairs to go to bed." Or, "I feel weak and I am having trouble opening jars." That will help your HCP focus much more quickly.

### Generalized weakness.
How you feel:
- Fatigued, weak, listless, no energy

Other indicators:
- Often associated with another illness (such as a cold) or condition (such as anemia or lack of sleep)

### Muscle-related weakness.
- Unable to do specific tasks due to lack of specific muscle strength
- May or may not be related to an illness

## COMMON TYPES OF DIZZINESS

When we talk to someone who uses the word "dizzy," we're trying to identify one of three things: are you lightheaded, do you have a condition called vertigo, or are you, well, dizzy?

### Lightheaded.
Most of the time, people get lightheaded when their blood pressure drops. Something as simple as standing up too fast when you normally have low blood pressure can cause your blood pressure to drop. Or, your blood pressure may be low because you're dehydrated or recently started taking a new medicine to lower your blood pressure.

You can also get lightheaded when your head feels stuffy from a bad cold or allergies. The key to identifying lightheadedness is that you don't feel like the room is spinning, you don't feel numbness or tingling on one side of your body, and you do feel better if you lie down.

How you feel:
- Like you're gong to pass out (also called feeling "woozy")
- Better when you lie down
- Not nauseated, and no vomiting
- Hearing not affected
- Able to carry daily activities

## Vertigo.

Vertigo is to dizzy what the equator is to warm. Vertigo is caused by an inner ear problem and is not related to blood pressure.

People with true vertigo feel motion when they are still and often describe the sensation as spinning, rotating, or whirling. They may fall over if they try to stand up and walk because they are trying to compensate for motion they sense, but that isn't actually there.

When you were a kid, did you ever sit on a swing and have someone turn you around in a circle, twisting the ropes so that you got spun around like a top as they unwound? Feeling like that when you're flat on the floor is vertigo. Vertigo can be completely disabling. You're not reading this yourself if you are currently experiencing vertigo.

How you feel:
- Sense of motion when you are still
- Lying down does not make you feel better; lying flat on your back can make the sensation worse
- Nauseated and vomiting
- Hearing may be lost in one ear, or there can be ringing or buzzing in the ear
- You can barely walk or move around without falling

## Dizzy.

That brings us back to dizzy, which, after you consider the more precise terms of lightheadedness and vertigo, is fairly uncommon. If you don't fit into those two categories and still feel unsteady, we can call that dizzy.

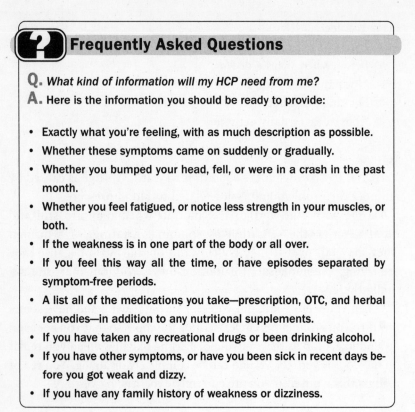

## Frequently Asked Questions

Q. *What kind of information will my HCP need from me?*

A. Here is the information you should be ready to provide:

- Exactly what you're feeling, with as much description as possible.
- Whether these symptoms came on suddenly or gradually.
- Whether you bumped your head, fell, or were in a crash in the past month.
- Whether you feel fatigued, or notice less strength in your muscles, or both.
- If the weakness is in one part of the body or all over.
- If you feel this way all the time, or have episodes separated by symptom-free periods.
- A list all of the medications you take—prescription, OTC, and herbal remedies—in addition to any nutritional supplements.
- If you have taken any recreational drugs or been drinking alcohol.
- If you have other symptoms, or have you been sick in recent days before you got weak and dizzy.
- If you have any family history of weakness or dizziness.

## TECHNICALLY SPEAKING ...

Vertigo is usually related to problems in the ear. A complex system deep in your ear called the labyrinth (LAB-uh-rinth) is responsible for your sense of balance and your ability to determine your body's position in relation to your surroundings. When you get motion sickness, for example, it's because this system gets completely overloaded by the nearly continuous movement of your body—typically on a boat or airplane. The nerves located in the labyrinth send scrambled messages to your brain, which brings on nausea and even vomiting. Motion sickness remedies work by decreasing the inner ear's sensitivity to small amounts of motion, so you're less likely to get sick. If the labyrinth becomes inflamed, you can develop vertigo.

Another condition that affects this balance system is Ménière (men-YEAR) disease. No one knows exactly what causes Ménière disease, so treatments are directed at managing the symptoms. It can range from occasional episodes to such frequent balance problems that it interferes with daily activities.

## NURSE'S WISDOM

- Don't try to drive or to "operate heavy machinery" if you are experiencing lightheadedness, vertigo, or dizziness.
- Don't starve yourself if you are trying to lose weight; low blood sugar can cause these symptoms.
- If you have true vertigo, it may be easier for you to crawl on the floor to get to the bathroom, for example, than trying to walk when your symptoms are most severe. Crawling may seem strange but it will reduce the risk of falls and injuries.
- Get up slowly if you've been lightheaded. If you're lying down, first move to a sitting position for one to two minutes, then stand up *slowly*.
- Keep drinking fluids; dehydration can make you feel weak and dizzy.
- Know that drowsiness is a common side effect of medications used to treat vertigo.

## SELF-CARE

The best advice is to take it easy based on how you feel. Since weakness and dizziness are usually associated with another problem, take care of that. Protect yourself from injury by sitting or lying down if you are very unsteady.

## LISTEN UP!

HCPs are not police officers. If you feel weak or dizzy, it is essential that you are honest about any recreational drug use and about the amount of alcohol you drink. Lying or withholding that information can delay proper care and can hurt you in the long run.

## RASHES AND ITCHES

### NURSE'S NOTE

Since an entire book could easily be devoted to rashes and itching problems, we will cover the basics here as well as how to determine when self-care is appropriate, when you need to go to the ER, or when you need to see your HCP. This section covers common skin problems as well as itching caused by anal conditions and vaginal yeast infections.

OTC hemorrhoid and rectal treatments are popular because people are embarrassed to talk to their HCP about that part of the body, but you're not alone; 75% of Americans will have a hemorrhoid at least once in their lives. However, rectal bleeding can be caused by something very simple, such as a hemorrhoid, or it can signal growths in the colon that need to be checked out. If you notice bleeding for the first time on your underwear, on toilet tissue, or in the toilet, get it checked.

Once a woman had has a vaginal yeast infection, she will know if she gets another. That is the theory behind making the drugs that treat these infections available without a prescription. However, yeast infections can occur at the same time as bacterial infections, and it may be difficult to determine if a yeast or bacterial infection is causing your symptoms without looking at the discharge under a microscope. Talk with your HCP about whether self-treatment of a presumed yeast infection is appropriate for you, or if you're better off having an exam for a more accurate diagnosis when you have symptoms.

### GET THEE TO THE ER

You need to go to the ER if you have a rash all over your body (not limited to just one area, such as your arm) and one or more of the following:

- A fever over about 101 degrees Fahrenheit.
- Weakness and fatigue.
- A stiff neck and headache, and normal room light hurts your eyes.
- The rash has come on suddenly, with raised welts and itchiness, and you're starting to have trouble breathing or you feel as if your throat is closing up.
- Other symptoms that come on at the same time as the rash or shortly thereafter (for example, within a day), such as vomiting, diarrhea, headache, dizziness, or confusion.

Do not go to the ER unless you are very sick and cannot get hold of your HCP, if you think you may have one of the traditional childhood illnesses such as chicken pox, German measles (rubella), measles, or mumps, even as an adult. These are highly contagious diseases, and if you go to the ER, you'll have to be isolated from other patients so you don't infect someone else. If you do need to go to the ER, have a companion drive or at least go with you. Before you go in, have the companion run in and talk to the nurse first.

## CALL YOUR HEALTH CARE PROVIDER

- If you have any rash or itchy condition that does not improve after a week of self-care.
- If you have any kind of sore that doesn't heal within three weeks.
- If you have a red, warm area near a break in the skin, with increasing pain, swelling, redness, red streaks, or pus-like drainage. All of these signs may indicate that you have an infection.
- If you have little pinpoint dots or bruises and you are not sick.
- If you have pinpoint dots or bruises that came on at the same time as a fever and other symptoms, get to the ER right away.
- If you have painful—not itchy—red blisters that typically form a pattern, usually on just one side of the body.

■ If you have a rash with joint pain.
■ If you notice an abnormality in your skin that doesn't itch or hurt or spread, but is a change in a mole or birthmark you already had or one that meets the ABCD criteria:

A—Asymmetry (if you put a line down the middle of the abnormality, it is not the same on both sides).
B—Border is irregular.
C—Color is often unusual and may include variable shades of brown, tan, black, red, blue or white.
D—Diameter is larger than a pencil eraser.

■ If you have spots of rectal bleeding that you have never had before.
■ If you cannot move your bowels because your anal discomfort is so severe.
■ If you have fever, abdominal pain, and a vaginal discharge.

## COMMON TYPES OF SKIN RASHES THAT ITCH

### Contact dermatitis.

Contact dermatitis is caused by coming in contact with something that makes your skin irritated or to which you are allergic. The rash often appears in a pattern that matches your exposure; for example, if you are sensitive to the elastic in underwear, you may have a ring around your waist.

Contact dermatitis is also the name given to the reaction you'll get if you come into contact with poison ivy, oak, or sumac. In this case, you will have been outside and the rash will often be in a streaky pattern that matches how the leaves brushed against your skin.

How you feel:
■ Pain (irritation) or itchiness (allergic) in the area
■ Not sick

Other indicators:
- Rarely, the skin will blister and weep

Nurse's orders:
- Try to identify the substance to which you're allergic (or the irritant) by process of elimination, and minimize exposure
- Apply cold compresses to the affected area
- Use anti-inflammatory ointment or cream, prescription or OTC

## Eczema.
Eczema is also called atopic dermatitis, which is another term used for people who are particularly sensitive to allergens and irritants.

How you feel:
- Itchiness on the skin
- Not sick

Other indicators:
- Skin is red and sometimes flaky
- May have bumps

Nurse's orders:
- Take brief showers in warm—not hot—water
- Pat—don't rub—skin dry and apply an unscented moisturizer before skin is completely dry to help hold in moisture
- Use mild, unscented soaps for bathing and laundry
- Take an OTC or prescription antihistamine if itching interferes with daily activities (particularly sleep) and/or prescription creams or ointments from your HCP

## COMMON TYPES OF SKIN RASHES THAT DON'T PARTICULARLY ITCH

### Rosacea.

This is a condition characterized by redness, particularly on the face, initially resembling windburn. It affects 14 million people, typically of Northern European descent, who have fair skin.

How you feel:
- In early stages, you seem to blush easily with persistent redness in the center of the face—for example, on your forehead, nose, cheeks, or chin
- As rosacea progresses, the redness stays, and can look like you got a little too much sun
- You may also have bumps and little pimples as well as dry, irritated eyes
- Not sick

Nurse's orders:
- See a dermatologist for firm diagnosis and appropriate prescription(s) for your skin type
- Never put OTC or prescription anti-inflammatory ointment or cream on your face without the specific instruction of your HCP after you've been examined: this self-treatment can make rosacea worse
- Be especially careful about protecting your skin from the sun
- Use mild, unscented soaps and moisturizers on your skin

### Rashes signaling other diseases.

Some conditions start with a rash before or at the same time other symptoms appear. These include Lyme disease, Rocky Mountain Spotted Fever, and many rheumatic diseases including forms of arthritis and rheumatic fever. While you may read about a characteristic bull's-eye rash with Lyme disease, for example, a specific type of rash is not required for diagnosis, so you don't have to worry about whether your rash pattern "matches" the textbook or not.

How you feel:

- Sick; depending on the illness, you may have joint pain, fever, headache, or fatigue
- Rash does not itch

Other indicators:

- You've been in a place where you may have been bitten by a tick; note that the ticks that carry this disease are tiny—about the size of a period in a sentence—so they are very easy to miss

Nurse's orders:

- Call your HCP, and if you feel very sick and can't get a response, go to the ER

## COMMON CAUSES OF ITCHING WITH OR WITHOUT A SKIN RASH

### Fungal infections.

Two common places where you can get fungal infections of the skin are the feet, where the infection is commonly called athlete's foot, or the groin, where it is commonly called jock itch. For ease of organization here, we'll also include the female equivalent of jock itch, vaginal yeast infections.

How you feel:

- Intense itching in the affected area
- Redness, either caused by scratching or by irritation from the initial infection
- Not sick

How you feel with a vaginal yeast infection:

- Severe itching of the vagina and the external genitalia
- Pain during intercourse or when urine flows across irritated skin

Other indicators of a vaginal yeast infection:

■ An odorless white discharge that looks like cottage cheese may appear
■ Yeast is more likely if these symptoms occur during or shortly after you've taken antibiotics for another condition

Nurse's orders:

■ Keep the area dry
■ Wear cotton clothing and leather footwear that breathe instead of ones made from synthetics
■ Use an OTC antifungal agent to start, or use prescription medication from your HCP

**Hemorrhoids and anal itching.**
Hemorrhoids are enlarged veins around the anus. Anal itching can also occur if the anal area is not cleaned after a bowel movement (cleaning is painful with hemorrhoids), and is caused by fungal infections and cracks in the skin around the anus.

How you feel:

■ Itchy and with a burning sensation, sometimes intense, in the anal area
■ Pain with bowel movements

Other indicators:

■ Small amounts of red blood on toilet tissue, underwear, or in the toilet after a bowel movement

Nurse's orders:

■ See your HCP for a diagnosis since you won't be able to see the area yourself
■ Take OTC remedies once cleared by your HCP

## ❓ Frequently Asked Questions

Q. *Will ointments and creams burn when I apply them?*

A. It depends on your skin condition and your sensitivity. You might feel a stinging or burning initially, but if the medicine continues to cause discomfort, wash it off, stop using it, and check with your HCP.

Q. *Can antifungal medicines be used to prevent jock itch?*

A. They're not meant as preventive medicine; drying powders containing cornstarch may help reduce the risk you'll get it. Your HCP may recommend you continue to apply the medicine for a few weeks even after the rash clears up to reduce the risk it will come back.

Q. *Is a vaginal yeast infection contagious?*

A. No, it is not considered a sexually transmitted disease.

Q. *Does it matter if I use ointment, gel, or suppositories for anal treatments?*

A. It's really personal preference. If you find one form or product gives you better relief than another, use what works!

## NURSE'S WISDOM

Poison ivy and other allergic rashes are not contagious. The rash may blister and weep, but that fluid does not contain any allergens. The fluid is much like plasma, the watery component of blood.

Depending on your degree of sensitivity, you can be exposed to the chemical on the poison ivy leaf that causes the skin reaction, for example, by brushing up against the leaf, by touching clothing that has touched the leaf, or by petting your dog who has gotten the leaf's chemical on its fur. If you are highly allergic, you can develop a rash with no recollection of how you might have been exposed. Poison ivy is particularly dangerous if it is burned and you get

## Did You Know?

Most women consider themselves experts when it comes to diagnosing their own vaginal yeast infections. Yet, the symptoms of vaginal discharge, burning, itching, or painful intercourse are caused by yeast only about 25% of the time.

When medication to treat yeast infections switched from prescription-only to OTC, their sales skyrocketed. But there wasn't a corresponding epidemic of yeast infections. Research showed that women were misdiagnosing themselves—they made the correct self-diagnosis only 25% to 30% of the time. If your self-care does not relieve your symptoms within a week or you're not positive about your diagnosis, see your HCP for a quick exam and precise diagnosis.

smoke that contains the chemical in your eyes or throat. This can result in a serious reaction that requires a visit to your HCP, or in the case of your eyes, to your ophthalmologist or the ER.

- If you have dry skin, baby it. Buying soaps and other hygiene products designed for babies may be your best bet because they are less likely to have fragrances, alcohol, and other ingredients that can irritate sensitive skin.
- Other products that are designed for dry skin and recommended by dermatologists include Cetaphil, Eucerin, Aveeno for sensitive skin, and Oil of Olay products. Always look for products designed for sensitive skin, and check the label to see that fragrance or alcohol is not one of the first ingredients on the list. You may need to do some trial and error to see which product agrees with your skin.
- Give your dry skin a rest; there is no law that says you have to shower every day, and certainly not more than once a day.
- Trim your fingernails so if you scratch in your sleep, a sharp edge on a nail doesn't damage your skin.

■ Protect your hands, particularly if you live with dry heat in the wintertime. Wear gloves whenever you're doing activities that will get your hands wet or expose them to detergents or chemicals.

■ Many women with red faces first go to their favorite cosmetic counter to buy a product to get rid of or cover the redness, not knowing it could be rosacea. And today, many of the upscale skin creams have low levels of hydrocortisone in them. The person behind the counter may recommend the "anti-redness" cream, and you may not realize you're applying an OTC medication to your face. See your HCP or dermatologist for a diagnosis before you do anything to treat or cover a red face.

■ A vicious cycle often develops in people with hemorrhoids: it begins with constipation that requires straining during bowel movements. This straining displaces a vein that becomes a hemorrhoid. and becomes hemorrhoid. Then, the pain from the hemorrhoid makes a bowel movement painful, so stool is held. Stool that remains in the lower colon dries out, making it even harder and more difficult to expel.

■ Itching typically occurs because it is painful to clean the anal area. Use a local anesthetic first, and then use medicated pads to cleanse the anal area after a bowel movement.

■ Reduce coffee intake as residue from coffee beans can irritate the anal area.

■ Sometimes, the external itching is very uncomfortable and the worst symptom of a vaginal yeast infection. Even if you treat the infection in the vagina with a suppository or tablet, you can also buy a tube of cream and apply it to the external genital skin for symptom relief. (Keep the cream in the fridge for extra relief.)

■ To reduce moisture, men and women can set a blow-dryer on low, and direct it toward the genital area from about 18 inches away after showering and before dressing.

■ Whether itching is vaginal or anal, stick with plain white toilet paper without dyes or fragrances.

■ Always wash underwear in hot water to kill organisms that

can cause infection or irritation regardless of washing instructions. Plain white cotton fabric is best.

## SELF-CARE

### Contact dermatitis:

■ If you think you have come in contact with poison ivy or one of its botanical cousins, wash thoroughly with soap and water to get the substance that causes the allergic reaction off the skin. You may be able to beat a nasty rash!

■ Rub petroleum jelly on dry, scaly skin; at bedtime, you can put it on your hands and feet, then wear cotton gloves and socks while you sleep.

■ Soothe your skin with an oatmeal bath. You can buy a prepared powder, such as Aveeno Soothing Bath.

### Fungal infections:

■ For athlete's foot, wash your feet daily and dry between the toes so feet are completely dry before putting on cotton socks and natural leather footwear.

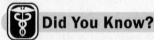 **Did You Know?**

Yes, it is true that Preparation H is a popular skin care product used with movie and television makeup because it reduces puffiness, dark circles, and small wrinkles around the eyes. However, the formulation has changed. It used to contain live yeast cell derivative (LYCD). Years ago, when the FDA required companies to show scientific proof of ingredients' effectiveness, there was no research on LYCD, so it was removed and an ingredient that shrinks blood vessels was added instead.

In Canada, however, LYCD remains in Preparation H, and two newer research studies in the United States have found it stimulates wound healing.

- Use an antifungal powder on your feet and in your shoes.
- Do not wear the same shoes two days in a row; it takes the fungus spores 24 hours to die.
- For jock itch, dust an antifungal powder on the genitals two or three times a day (creams can keep the area moist, and moist conditions help yeast grow).
- Wear fresh underwear every day and wash athletic supporters before each wearing.

### Hemorrhoids and anal itching:
- Cleanse your anal area with a damp washcloth or pre-moistened wipes; baby wipes are ideal.
- Eat a well-balanced diet to reduce constipation and the need for straining while having a bowel movement.
- Wear cotton underpants.

### Vaginal yeast infections:
- Wear only all-cotton underpants (the cotton panel is not enough); stay away from pantyhose and tight pants of any fabric.
- Do not sit in wet bathing suits or exercise clothing; change as soon as you are finished with your activities.

## OTC REMEDIES: SKIN CONDITIONS

Do not use any of these for more than 7 days unless specifically instructed by your HCP to use for a longer time.

### Antibiotics.
Bacitracin and a combination of neomycin, polymyxin B, and bacitracin help prevent skin bacterial infections. Apply to a cut or scrape to reduce infection risk. Apply to stitches only if instructed by the HCP. Infection will delay healing of cuts and scrapes. Some antibiotic creams and ointments are now combined with a numbing ingredient to reduce pain.

## Antifungal.

Clotrimazole, ketoconazole, and tolnaftate come in many formulations, including creams, lotions, powders, and gels. Use them to treat fungal skin infections including athlete's foot, jock itch and ringworm. Undecyclenic acid is an older drug that is not as common, but may be tried if the others don't clear up the skin.

## Anti-inflammatory.

Hydrocortisone is available as a cream, lotion, or ointment and can be used to treat rashes, itching, and skin irritation. Never use it on the face or neck, and if your condition is not significantly improved after seven days of use, see your HCP to determine if you need a prescription-strength drug instead.

## Itch relief.

Calamine is the mother of all anti-itch medicines, particularly for rashes caused by poison ivy and its cousins. It helps dry the oozing and weeping that goes with those rashes. It is now available in a combination with other ingredients that will soothe and numb the skin.

## OTC REMEDIES: HEMORRHOIDS AND ANAL ITCHING

Remedies for hemorrhoid discomfort and anal itching contain a combination of ingredients and come in a variety of forms includ-

### Did You Know?

The formulation of a skin product can moisturize or dry your skin. The formulations in order from least drying to most drying are: ointment >> cream >> lotion >> gel. Some experts say that the low doses in many ointments sold OTC are not strong enough to have a true therapeutic effect, and that prescription-strength medication is needed. Check with your HCP if you're not seeing much improvement with an OTC product.

ing creams, suppositories, ointments, gels, and medicated wipes. Use this guide if you can pinpoint what is causing the greatest discomfort, and choose the remedy with the ingredients that match your symptoms; otherwise, buy a small package and try more than one remedy to see what works for you. These are the medicinal ingredients; some products have additional ingredients to soothe the skin such as aloe.

### Mineral oil/petrolatum/shark liver oil.
These ingredients act to seal and protect irritated skin.

### Phenylephrine.
This ingredient shrinks blood vessels. Its use in hemorrhoid treatment is a bit controversial, however, because of the concern of rebound swelling, since that's what happens when phenylephrine is used as a decongestant nasal spray.

### Pramoxzine hydrochloride.
This is a local anesthetic in the same family as benzocaine, which can temporarily numb the area to relieve pain and itching.

### Witch hazel.
Witch hazel is an astringent that aids in wound healing (or dry, cracked skin), and reduces pain. This ingredient is most commonly sold as saturated pads for cleansing and moisturizing.

## OTC REMEDIES: VAGINAL YEAST INFECTIONS

Medicines in this category include butoconazole nitrate, clotrimazole, niconazole, and ticonazole. They come in different forms: cream that is put in the vagina with an applicator, vaginal tablets, or vaginal suppositories. For an uncomplicated yeast infection, they are all effective, and your choice may be based on medicine form, price, and convenience of dosing schedule.

## LISTEN UP!

The number of causes of rashes and itching is almost as varied as the number of people who experience these conditions. Try self-care, limit your exposure to irritants, and be sure to follow up with your HCP if you can't solve the problem on your own within a week or so.

# ■ COLD AND FEVER ■

## COUGH

### NURSE'S NOTE

As both an RN and a registered respiratory therapist, I am a cough expert. I can tell you dozens of fancy words to describe the mucus people hack up! Should you worry about your cough? Key aspects to focus on are whether the cough is new or has been going on for a long time, whether you feel sick when you get the cough, and whether you're coughing up anything.

### GET THEE TO THE ER

You should take a ride to the ER if:

■ You cough up blood.
■ You cough up pink, frothy mucus.
■ You cough and you are also very short of breath.
■ You suddenly start coughing and think you have something stuck in your throat.

## CALL YOUR HEALTH CARE PROVIDER

- If you have a cough that last two or more weeks, you don't feel sick, and can't readily identify a cause.
- If you have a new cough and are producing mucus that is green or yellow, has blood streaks, or looks like currant jelly.
- If you know you have been exposed to a potentially toxic gas or fumes (and you aren't going to the ER).
- If you develop a cough after starting a prescription for high blood pressure. (Don't stop taking the medicine before you check in.)
- If your chest feels tight when you cough, and the chest tightness and cough come and go.
- If your cough is worse after you eat a big meal or spicy foods, or is associated with burning or a bad taste in the back of your throat.
- If your cough is preventing you from sleeping.
- If you have true influenza and want to ask about antiviral medication. (It's a complicated decision, and the medication is not right for everyone.)
- If you have a cough and are sick for more than a few days, or you have a high fever and are very sick.

If you have a cough and any concerns, check in with your HCP. If a friend or loved one has developed a cough, encourage them not to ignore it and to at least call their HCP, too.

## INSIDER INFO

I have had hundreds of conversations with patients that went something like this:

PAT: So, how did you injure your wrist?
PATIENT: (cough, cough) I didn't have a chance to put salt down, and I (cough, cough) slipped on the ice.

PAT: Can you wiggle your fingers?

PATIENT: Yeah, but (cough, cough) it sure hurts like the dickens.

PAT: How long have you had that cough?

PATIENT: Cough? What cough?

After a while, people don't even notice they have a chronic cough. It has become part of them, like that funny twitch in their face. Family members often don't hear it any longer, either; they get used to it, like you get used to the street noise if you live in a city or the crickets that sing at night in warm weather out in the country.

Also, people who are afraid they have a lung disease may deny having a cough. One coughing patient told me, "I don't have a cough; I'm just clearing my throat." If you don't want to use the word cough, fine, but be aware it's still something to get checked out by your HCP.

## COMMON CAUSES OF COUGHS WHEN YOU FEEL SICK

Coughing is usually a reflex, stimulated by an irritation, intended to keep the breathing passages clear. A whole host of things can cause coughs: infections, allergies, the clearing of your breathing passages if you have swallowed something "the wrong way," lung diseases, medication side effects, the breathing in of something toxic or irritating, smoking, and the presence of fluid in the lungs. Coughing involves not only your chest muscles, but also your diaphragm (the main muscle of breathing) and tightening of your stomach (abdominal) muscles. That's one reason it's painful for people to cough after abdominal surgery. It also explains why you're usually sore if you've been coughing your head off as those muscles get quite a workout.

Some coughs are critical to keeping your breathing passages clear. Other coughs are just plain annoying—for example, a tickle in the back of your throat. Determining the difference helps guide proper care.

## Acute bronchitis.

This is an inflammation of the breathing passages—called bronchi (BRONK-eye)—usually because of a bacterial or viral infection. (Acute doesn't mean it's adorable; it means it is short rather than long term, also called chronic.) Acute bronchitis is the formal name for a cold that "goes to the chest." Cough and chest congestion typically start within a week of the cold. Acute bronchitis can also occur after exposure to a substance particularly irritating to your lungs.

How you feel:
- Sick but still able to go about your everyday activities
- Tightness in the chest, but not short of breath

Other indicators:
- Cough may produce green or yellow mucus
- Productive, wet cough that follows a cold or exposure to strong irritant
- Low fever, if any

Nurse's order:
- Practice self-care if viral infection
- Take prescription antibiotic only if bacterial infection

## Influenza.

There is only one flu—and you'll know when you have it. If you're not sure whether you have the flu, you don't. Influenza is a respiratory infection; there is no such thing as "stomach flu."

How you feel:
- Very sick—flat out in bed
- Severe body aches, headache
- May have sore throat
- Exhausted
- May or may not be short of breath

Other indicators:
- Sudden onset (within hours from feeling fine to being flat-out sick)
- High fever
- Dry cough

Nurse's order:
- Take OTC pain reliever to treat symptoms (unless there are complications)
- Get a flu shot every year
- Check with your HCP about whether anti-influenza medication is right for you once you are sick

## Pneumonia.

Unlike bronchitis, which affects only the breathing passages, pneumonia is a viral or bacterial infection that is in the lung tissue—the air sacs—itself. (There are other causes of pneumonia, but we'll leave those to the specialists.) "Walking pneumonia" is a common description for a viral infection, or a specific type of infection called Mycoplasma (MY-coe-PLAZ-muh). Serious pneumonia and its complications are more common in people over age 65, those who smoke, those who have chronic diseases such as emphysema or HIV, or those taking chemotherapy that suppresses the immune system. In these people, pneumonia can be life-threatening.

### Viral pneumonia

How you feel:
- Sick, but usually still able to carry out your everyday activities (but at a slower pace)
- May have a sore throat, aches and pains, and the like

Other indicators:
- Usually low fever
- Usually not short of breath
- Cough for a week or less
- Cough up green or yellow mucus

Nurse's order:
- Don't take antibiotics
- Treat symptoms with OTC cough or pain remedies

### Bacterial pneumonia
How you feel:
- Usually quite ill and not able to carry out your usual daily routine
- Pain in the chest with a deep breath may occur

Other indicators:
- Usually high fever and chills
- Cough for a week or less
- Cough up green or yellow mucus
- May be short of breath

Nurse's order:
- Take antibiotic prescription from HCP
- Get a pneumonia vaccine if you are over age 65 or are at high risk for bacterial pneumonia

**Tuberculosis.**
Tuberculosis, or TB, has made a bit of a comeback because more people are living with impaired immune systems that put them at risk for uncommon infections. "TB infection" means you have the bacteria in your body, but you are not actively sick. Your skin test will be positive. "TB disease" is the term used when you're sick.

Chances of your having TB are remote unless you have traveled to a country where a lot of people have TB, or if you work with people who are at risk for TB, such as in prisons, homeless shelters, ERs, and the like.

How you feel:
- May or may not feel sick
- Usually not short of breath

Other indicators:

- Positive skin test
- Exposure to other people who have (or are at high risk for) TB
- Wet, productive cough that lasts for weeks to months
- Cough may have bloody streaks in it
- Night sweats
- Weight loss

Nurse's order:

- Take long-term antibiotics as prescribed by your HCP

## COMMON CAUSES OF COUGHS WHEN YOU DON'T FEEL SICK

### Postnasal drip.

This is the most common cause of coughs. Our noses and throats produce mucus all the time—normally 1 to 2 quarts per day! Postnasal drip is the feeling that this mucus is collecting in the back of your throat. Typically this happens when your mucus production factory is working overtime, because you have a cold, allergies, are breathing cold air, eating spicy foods, or experiencing hormonal changes. This drip, drip, drip of mucus can be irritating and give you a dry or wet cough. Postnasal drip is worse when you're lying down or sleeping and not swallowing as often.

### Smoker's cough.

Cigarette smoke is an irritant. Irritants stimulate the cough reflex. The end.

There are two lung diseases caused primarily by long-term cigarette smoking: chronic bronchitis and emphysema. The most recent national guidelines suggest that we stop calling them two different diseases and group them together under the name "chronic obstructive pulmonary disease," or COPD. In COPD, changes in the lungs over time (decades) cause blockage of the breathing passages, which triggers a cough. A COPD cough is different from a smoker's cough in that it occurs in people who've been smoking for a long time. But either way, if you smoke and you have a dry or wet cough, your body is trying to tell you the smoke is irritating and damaging your throat and lungs. It's not a normal "side effect."

## Asthma.

Many people think asthma equals wheezing. But for many people, a dry cough is the only sign of asthma. If you've developed a cough with no clear cause, you don't smoke, and you don't feel sick, make an appointment with your HCP for an evaluation to see if you may have asthma.

## Allergies and irritants.

You can develop a dry cough with allergies. You'll probably also have sneezing; watery, itchy eyes; and a runny nose. Inhaling irritants such as smoke, air pollution, fumes, or other particles (in the workplace, for example) can trigger a cough, as can irritants in the home such as dust or pet dander. With this kind of cough, you'll stop coughing when you're not exposed to the irritant.

## Acid reflux.

Acid reflux can also be referred to by its fancy name, gastroesophageal (GAS-troh-ess-OFF-uh-gee-ul) reflux disease, or GERD.

 **Frequently Asked Questions**

Q. *Can a cough be a side effect of medication?*
A. Yes. In fact, a category of drugs used to treat high blood pressure, called ACE inhibitors, causes a dry, hacking cough in about 10% of the people who take them. The cough doesn't cause any harm, however. Whether the drug needs to be stopped usually depends on how annoyed you (or other people around you) are by the cough. If you develop a cough while taking one of these medicines, don't stop without checking with your HCP.

## 🩺 Did You Know?

A nursing research study from Oregon Health Sciences University tracked the types of foods that triggered asthma reactions, which often start with a cough. Of 914 patients ages 3 to 55, 45% reported adverse reactions to milk, red wine, eggs, chocolate, and peanuts. And patients who had food reactions were more likely to have been hospitalized than the people who did not report food reactions. You might want to keep a diary of what you've eaten if you have periodic episodes of coughing without an obvious cause.

With GERD, acid that should stay in the stomach backwashes into the esophagus (the tube between the throat and the stomach) and the back of the throat. The acid irritates the back of your throat and makes you cough. This kind of cough is more common after lying down, particularly after a full night of sleep.

### Annoying tickle.

It's not a fancy medical term, but we all know what it is, right? A tickle can occur when your throat is dry. It can also be a stimulus to cough "leftover" from a cold or sinus infection, or it can be allergy related. The key with this dry cough is that it doesn't protect or clear your airway—it's just annoying.

## NURSE'S WISDOM

- Limit all particles in the air that can be irritating and worsen your cough (regardless of cause), particularly sprays around your face. For example, instead of sprays, use roll-on or cream deodorant, hair gels, or liquid perfumes. Also avoid using powders that can create a cloud of dust.
- Think about your household products, too. Instead of sprays, use special dusting cloths, solid air fresheners, or cleansing wipes.

■ Vacuum regularly with a machine that has (at minimum) a two-stage filter; three-stage is best. Choose a vacuum with a HEPA filter system; it's the same type of filter used in masks we wear for protection in the hospital. If your vacuum doesn't have these features, you'll simply push dust, dirt, and allergens into the air rather than sucking them up.

■ Consider hiring help (or ask a friend or family member for help) if cleaning your home or doing yard work makes you cough for a few days.

■ If outdoor allergens bother you, don't dry clothes, towels, or bedding outside on the line; it will just bring the problems from the outside indoors.

■ Wear a mask to protect yourself from inhaling allergens and irritants if all else fails.

■ For acid reflux, place thick phone books or special bed risers of the same size beneath the legs to raise the head of the bed about six inches. If you're away from home and can't raise your bed, lie on your left side. That will keep your esophagus higher than your stomach, so gravity will help keep acid where it belongs.

■ If you have acid reflux and a cough, don't bend over to lift; instead, bend at the knees. Don't wear tight clothing around your waist. Both of these can push acid up out of your stomach.

■ Breathe in steam to soothe your cough. You can sit on a chair in your bathroom with the door closed and turn the shower on hot. *Do not get in the shower;* instead, breathe in the steam the hot water creates.

## SELF-CARE

### Coughs:

■ Drink, drink, drink. Having plenty of fluids in your system keeps mucus thin so you can cough it out. It also keeps your throat moist, which will help reduce that annoying tickle-type cough.

- Get as much rest as you can. Coughs are very physically demanding, and they often interrupt sleep. You may not awaken, but coughing can nudge you out of the deepest phases of sleep that are most restorative. Good quality sleep also strengthens your immune system.
- Don't smoke.
- Stay away from irritants you can inhale. If the outdoor air quality if poor, stay indoors.
- If your home is dry, use a humidifier to get the relative humidity to at least 30%.
- If your cough is dry and irritating, choose an OTC cough medicine (with an ingredient such as dextromethorphan) that will suppress the cough so you can sleep.
- Do *not* try to suppress a productive (wet) cough. Use an expectorant such as guaifenesin to help loosen mucus so it's easier to cough up.
- Put very warm compresses on your chest or back to relieve muscle pain from coughing.

## Asthma:
- If you are having a coughing spasm and having trouble catching your breath, consciously be calm.
- Sit still or lie on your side in a fetal position.
- Try to breathe in through your nose so any irritants can be filtered.
- Try to get your cough settled down before using inhaled medicine so you don't cough it right back out.

## Allergies and irritants:
- If you're allergic to pollen or mold spores, monitor the counts. Stay indoors if counts are high.
- Keep a cough diary to see if you can make associations between places you've been or foods you've eaten and increased coughing.

## Bacterial acute bronchitis, pneumonia, or TB:

- Be sure to take every antibiotic pill—even if you feel cured and half of the pills remain—so that you'll kill of all the bacteria.
- TB requires antibiotics for a very long time, at least four to six months. If you stop early, TB bacteria can become much, much harder to kill.

## Acid reflux:

- Elevate your head during sleep; it's best to actually raise the head of the bed on 4- to 6-inch blocks. Otherwise, use a lot of pillows or a wedge under the bottom sheet to prop yourself up from the waist.
- Eat dinner many hours before going to bed.
- Don't eat anything right before going to bed.
- Lose weight if you're overweight.
- Use OTC medicines such as antacids and acid blockers *until* you can see your HCP for a work-up and diagnosis, but *not instead* of a visit.

## COUGH REMEDIES

If you need cough medicine, buy single-ingredient cough medicine. What's the difference? Let me explain.

Take one popular cough medicine called "flu syrup," which contains the following *per dose:* acetaminophen (pain reliever) 640 mg, chlorpheniramine maleate (antihistamine) 4 mg, dextromethorphan (cough suppressant) 20 mg, and pseudoephedrine (decongestant) 60 mg. Is that what is says on the label? No, and that's the problem. The label lists the number of milligrams for each ingredient in one teaspoon (5 mL). But the label also instructs you to take four teaspoons every four hours. Thus, in order to determine exactly how much of each ingredient you'll be taking, you need to multiply the numbers on the label by four—the four teaspoons the label recommends as the proper dose. Confusing? You bet. Who wants to pull out a calculator when you're sick? But if you don't do the math, you may think you need to take supplemental acetaminophen or anti-histamine or decongestant, which could lead to an unintentional overdose.

And what about the medication itself? If you truly have the flu, you may need an expectorant that keeps the mucus moving, not a cough suppressant. Do you need an antihistamine? Are you allergic to the flu? Hardly. If you're coughing up mucus, antihistamines will actually dry the mucus, making it harder for you to cough it out. But they're often added to multisymptom products to make you drowsy and offset the decongestant's "hyper" side effect. Which brings us to the decongestant. Do you need it? Only if your nose is plugged up and you can't breathe. If you can skip it, you won't have any "hyper" side effects that need to be counteracted with the drowsy side effect of the antihistamine that you probably don't need in the first place. See what I mean?

If you have aches and pains, buy a pain reliever. For your cough, buy either an expectorant or cough suppressant and go from there. Talk with you pharmacist or HCP for advice specific to your cough.

Cough medicines are pretty simple. There are two main OTC cough medicines: guaifenesin, an expectorant, which thins the mucus, and dextromethorphan, a cough suppressant, which reduces the urge to cough and is considered to be as effective as low-dose morphine. Menthol and camphor are not technically cough sup-pressants. They soothe the membranes in the nose and throat that, when irritated, make you cough. So lozenges or cough drops with these ingredients may be helpful. Use these OTC medicines for short-term coughs brought on by a mild infection only; for other coughs, use only if recommended by your HCP.

## ✚ When to Consider

**Expectorant:**
- Loosens thick mucus produced during a respiratory infection such as bronchitis, a cold, or sinus infection so the mucus can be coughed out.

**Cough suppressant (reduce cough):**
- Reduces coughing by making the cough center in the brain less sensitive.
- Quiet a cough that interferes with sleep.
- Reduce a dry cough that does not produce mucus and wears you out.

## ⊘ Do Not Use

- For a cough that has lasted more than a week.
- For a cough if you have asthma, are a smoker, or have any other lung disease such as emphysema or chronic bronchitis (also called COPD).
- A combination of a cough suppressant and an expectorant—why would you want to suppress a cough when you are loosening mucus? Choose one or the other.

## REMEDIES TO STOP SMOKING

If you're reading this because you've made the decision to stop smoking, or you're even thinking about kicking the habit, congratulations! Now that nicotine replacement therapy is available OTC, you can wean yourself off that drug. It's never too late; I am so proud of my mother who used patches to quit smoking a few years after her 70th birthday! Only 3% of people who go cold turkey are still smoke free six months later. If you combine nicotine replacement therapy with a program of some sort to help you overcome your habit, the average success rate doubles.

To help you deal with the habit aspect, GlaxoSmithKline and Pfizer each have a customized quitting support program that's free when you buy their nicotine replacement product. (See Web Resources, p. 303) You can also get information about the programs at the pharmacy where you buy the products.

The American Lung Association has a program called Freedom From Smoking. It is also online, or you can call your local chapter for information and materials. Many local chapters provide nicotine replacement products for free (often with the Great American Smokeout in November each year) or they subsidize the cost for people who join the program. Many states' Medicaid programs will cover the cost, and many employers offer smoking cessation programs at no cost.

There are many forms of nicotine replacement therapy, so you can choose the one you're most comfortable with.

### Patch.

This is a sticky square you put on your skin in an area without hair. You put it on in the morning, and it releases nicotine gradually during the day. You can choose either a 16-hour or 24-hour patch; some people have trouble sleeping if they leave the patch on, but others find wearing the patch through the night helps offset that morning craving. You can experiment and see what works best for you.

### Gum.

This is more like smoking. You can take a piece of gum and put it in your mouth at the times you would have a cigarette. You bite into the gum and then "park" it between your cheek and gum so the nicotine is absorbed through the lining of your mouth. The instructions recommend using the gum on a regular schedule, and you have to be careful not to chew more than the recommended daily maximum dose.

### Lozenge.

This form is recommended if you have a cigarette within 30 minutes of awakening.

### Spray nicotine and inhalers.

These are available by prescription only. They have the potential for abuse because the level of nicotine in your blood gets higher faster, and it's easy to increase the dose and stay hooked on nicotine.

## ➕ When to Consider

- Use nicotine replacement therapy to reduce physical withdrawal symptoms when you successfully quit smoking.

## 🚫 Do Not Use

- You absolutely, positively cannot smoke cigarettes or chew tobacco when you are using the patch. An overdose of nicotine can cause a heart attack.
- Do not try to adjust the nicotine dose of a patch by cutting it. It doesn't work that way. The nicotine is formulated in the patch to be gradually released over time; if you cut the patch, that time-release system could be damaged and you could get too much nicotine or none at all.
- Be very careful about how you discard a used patch. There will still be nicotine present, and it could be poisonous to children or animals.

## LISTEN UP!

The bottom line is that a cough is not normal. If you have a cough without an identifiable cause, you need to have it checked out. If you decide to take cough medicine, search the shelves and carefully read the labels to find the ingredient that's right for the type of cough you have. Remember that antihistamines can dry out mucus, so think twice before choosing an antihistamine if you have a productive cough.

# STUFFY OR RUNNY NOSE

## NURSE'S NOTE

Sometimes I feel like the only person on the earth who's blessed not to have sinus trouble. But that could be because self-diagnosis of sinusitis is often off the mark. Sinusitis is a very specific diagnosis, and antibiotics are not a must. In fact, using antibiotics for sinus infections assumed (but not proven) to be bacteria has led to an increase in what's called "resistant" bacteria—stronger bacteria that are harder to kill with everyday antibiotics. In addition, your symptoms may be complicated or caused by an allergy that makes your nose stuffy.

As with ear infections, don't try to get a diagnosis and treatment over the phone for what seems to be a sinus problem. In fact, between one-half and two-thirds of people with so-called sinus symptoms do *not* have a bacterial infection. I know it's not always easy to get an appointment or convenient to squeeze one into your day. But it's important; experts are now strongly encouraging more careful examinations before antibiotics are prescribed.

## GET THEE TO THE ER

- If you have sinusitis, your face becomes swollen, and your vision is impaired or blurry.
- If you have a nosebleed in which the blood runs down the back of your throat or comes out of both nostrils at the same time, or one that does not stop with basic self-care measures. Nosebleeds can be serious; don't hesitate to call 911.

## CALL YOUR HEALTH CARE PROVIDER

- If a cold seems to go away and then comes back with worsening congestion and pain; this pattern is more indicative of sinusitis.
- If symptoms of a cold don't go away in a week to ten days.
- If you also have a fever, are coughing up green mucus, or have other signs of a more serious condition.
- If you need to ask about alternative remedies for your stuffy nose because taking a decongestant makes you jittery or unable to sleep.

- If you have facial pain that doesn't go away.
- If you have allergy symptoms that self-care doesn't relieve.
- If you have recurrent anterior nosebleeds (described later in this section) without an obvious reason.
- If your HCP has prescribed aspirin therapy or anticoagulants such as Coumadin and you get anterior nosebleeds.

## INSIDER INFO

Truth is, a lot of people believe that an antibiotic prescription is their reward for the chore of visiting their HCP or going to an urgent care center. Many physicians would rather keep patients happy and provide the prescription rather than arguing, and I can't blame them. But the nose-cold-sinus bugs that make you feel awful are rarely caused by bacterial infections, so antibiotics won't work. As your mother told you, patience is a virtue. Don't demand an antibiotic prescription for the "instant cure"; instead, talk with your HCP about whether antibiotics are appropriate. You can save some money and avoid side effects that way, and an open discussion with your HCP never hurts.

## COMMON TYPES OF NASAL PROBLEMS

### Sinusitis.
Sinusitis is an inflammation of your sinuses, the air-filled chambers in your skull behind your nose and eyes. Sinusitis can be acute—a short-term problem—or chronic and longer term. Many things can set off this inflammation, including a viral or bacterial infection, allergies, or exposure to cold air.

Your HCP can diagnose acute sinusitis through a careful, targeted physical exam. If the diagnosis is in doubt, or if you've had symptoms for a long time, your HCP may collect drainage for a culture to see if bacteria grow, order sinus X rays or a head CT scan that shows the sinuses, or refer you to a specialist who may examine your sinuses with a special lighted scope.

### Viral sinusitis
How you feel:
- Stuffed or runny nose for more than a month
- Lousy with muscle aches, sore throat, and maybe facial pain or pressure

Other indicators:
- Recent exposure to a virus (such as the common cold)
- Thick drainage
- Decreased ability to taste or smell
- Symptoms getting worse rather than better
- Antihistamines have no effect

Nurse's order:
- Take OTC remedies to treat specific symptoms, such as: pain, congestion, and the like

### Bacterial sinusitis
How you feel:
- Stuffed or runny nose for more than a month
- Facial pain or pressure when you bend over from your waist to tie your shoes, for example (more prominent than body aches)

Other indicators:
- Recent exposure to a virus (such as the common cold)
- Thick green or yellow drainage from nose
- Decreased ability to taste or smell
- Symptoms getting worse rather than better
- Antihistamines have no effect

Nurse's order:
- Take an antibiotic as prescribed by your HCP

### Allergic sinusitis

How you feel:
- Stuffed or runny nose for more than a month
- Itchy, watery eyes
- Sneezing

Other indicators:
- Symptoms follow exposure to allergens
- Clear, watery drainage from nose
- Symptoms are staying about the same, not getting worse
- Antihistamines improve symptoms

Nurse's order
- Take OTC or prescription antihistamines

## Colds.

A cold is caused by a virus, which means you shouldn't take antibiotics unless you have some underlying condition that needs special care. As the old saying goes: If you treat a cold, it will typically last a week; without treatment, it will last about seven days. Colds are very contagious. Contrary to common belief, however, colds are not spread by people sneezing into the air. They are much more commonly spread by your hands. For example, you're a polite person and shake hands with people at a holiday party. Undoubtedly, someone will have a virus and will have touched his nose before he shakes your hand. If you then scratch or touch your nose, tag, you're it! And if you're run down from lack of sleep (who gets enough sleep, anyway?), a cold is just about 24 hours away.

A cold is generous, giving you multiple symptoms including a stuffy or runny nose, sore throat, headache, and fatigue.

## Allergies.

Allergies are characterized by a release of histamine in response to a substance your body has decided is potentially dangerous, even though it isn't. When that substance comes in contact with the mucous membranes in the nose, your body overreacts, causing the watery or stuffy nose, itchy eyes, and other symptoms such as feeling "foggy" that you're familiar with. When you get away from those substances, symptoms improve.

### Runny nose.

The fancy name for a runny nose is vasomotor rhinitis (vay-zo-MOtor rye-NY-tiss). With this condition, you'll have a runny nose with clear discharge, you won't feel sick, and you'll have no allergy symptoms (except occasional sneezing). There is no release of histamine, which happens in allergies, so antihistamines aren't indicated. Vasomotor rhinitis is more commonly associated with irritants and changes in temperature, such as going in or out of air conditioning on a hot day. I've had this for years. My approach? Pants with a pocket to hold my ever-present tissue.

### Nosebleed.

There are two types of nosebleed. One is the simple nosebleed that occurs when the nose is dry and irritated, or when the lining has been scraped as a finger is inserted into the nostril (a.k.a. nose picking). Blood comes out of the nostril when you're upright. This is called an *anterior* nosebleed because it comes from the *front* of the nose. The second type of nosebleed makes up only about 10% of all nosebleeds but is more serious. When bleeding comes from high up in the *back* of the nose, it's called a *posterior* nosebleed. Blood may not come out of the nostrils; it may only go down the back of the throat. Caused primarily by arteriosclerosis, high blood pressure that ruptures a blood vessel, or problems with blood clotting, posterior nosebleeds always need a visit to the ER.

## TECHNICALLY SPEAKING . . .

Sinuses—hollowed-out areas in your skull—are in your cheek area, forehead, and jaw. They are lined with a membrane similar to your

**? Frequently Asked Questions**

Q. *Why don't you consider my sinus headache a headache? My head hurts!*

A. Sinus pain occurs in the sinuses, which are located in the cheeks and the forehead. Sinus pain is more correctly a face ache rather than a headache, which is related to the scalp, blood vessels, and muscles in the head (for more about headaches, see page 3). Sinus pain occurs when the sinuses are swollen and congested, blocking the normal passage of muscus. The drainage is trapped, causing pressure and pain. You can have a headache and sinus pain, but they're not the same.

Q. *Can vitamins and minerals cure a cold?*

A. Remedies have been promoted to prevent or shorten the length of the common cold. Here's what reviews of the research have to say:

*Vitamin C.* There is no evidence that long-term daily supplements of vitamin C prevent colds. Symptoms may not last as long when you take relatively high doses during the illness, but no specific dose is recommended.

*Zinc.* There is no strong evidence that zinc lozenges shorten the length of a cold. Furthermore, many people have side effects such as mouth irritation, nausea, and diarrhea. More research is needed to evaluate the potential benefits versus the side effects.

*Echinacea.* It is nearly impossible to evaluate research on echinacea extracts because there are more than 200 different preparations on the market and the research does not compare "apples to apples." Overall, research studies report that echinacea probably helps prevent and treat colds, but again, no specific preparation or dose can be recommended.

nose lining. Contrary to popular belief, they are not designed just to make your life miserable. They make the skull lighter than if it were solid bone, they warm and humidify inhaled air, and they add to the tone and timbre of your voice.

## NURSE'S WISDOM

- When your sinuses are congested, you may be more comfortable if you prop yourself up on pillows to sleep. Gravity helps promote drainage.
- Don't choose OTC medicines because the box says "sinus" or "cold" or "allergy," choose by the ingredients.
- OTC pills don't usually stop a runny nose unless it's caused by an allergy.
- Use caution with decongestant nasal sprays. If used more than a few days, a phenomenon called rebound can occur, meaning the nasal congestion gets worse than it was before you used the spray. People then go back to using the spray, and a vicious cycle begins.
- Use warm compresses to ease sinus pain. To make warm compresses, moisten about ten washcloths with water, and then heat them in the microwave so they are hot, but not hot enough to burn you. Put them into a warm crockpot (or slow cooker) and close the lid after you take out the top washcloth. Apply it to your face. When it cools, take it off, put it at the bottom of the stack of washcloths in the crock-pot and then remove the one on top and apply it to your face. By the time you get through the stack, the cool ones you put on the bottom will be warm again, and you'll have a never-ending, very convenient supply. (You can use this tip anytime you need to apply moist heat for any reason.)
- To reduce your risk of catching a cold, don't shake hands during cold season. If you're at a party or business gathering, hold a drink (water with a twist of lime is my choice) in your right hand; when you meet someone, raise your glass and gesture as a greeting rather than shaking hands.
- Keep a bottle of hand sanitizer in your purse, briefcase, or glove compartment. You can put a few drops in your hands unobtrusively whenever you think of it to kill those germs.
- Keep the membranes inside your nose moist by putting a little

dab of petroleum jelly in each nostril at bedtime. (Just don't put your finger back in the jar after touching your nose or you'll contaminate the whole jar.)

■ If you have allergies, wash your hair before you go to bed. Particles in the air cling to your hair. If you don't wash your hair after you're home for the night, the particles in your hair will be transferred to your pillow and you'll breathe them in while you sleep.

■ Try to avoid substances to which you are allergic first, before you take medication.

■ Antihistamines dry out mucous membranes all over the body. This can lead to constipation; urinary problems; burning, dry eyes; dry mouth (long term can lead to dental problems); dry throat; and dry nose. If you take an antihistamine, be sure to drink plenty of water to offset drying side effects; suck on sugarless hard candy to minimize dry mouth.

■ Just because an antihistamine doesn't make you feel sleepy, it doesn't mean it can't cause other side effects or slow your reaction time.

■ If you're taking a sedating OTC antihistamine, you need to be very careful about taking any other medicine that can make you sleepy—and you shouldn't drink alcohol.

■ Reserve the sedating antihistamines for when you're home for the night, don't need to drive, and can go to bed if you get sleepy.

■ Resist the urge to take another medicine to offset the drowsy side effect of OTC antihistamines; this is often the theory behind multisymptom remedies.

## SELF-CARE

If you have any nose problem, don't smoke. It dries out the mucous membranes and will make a nose problem worse. Keep the humidity in your home at at least 30%. To measure indoor humidity, you can use a device called a humidity sensor (also known as a moisture meter, humidistat, or hygrometer). When you need to blow your nose, skip the handkerchief; use disposable tissues instead. To keep your nose from getting sore, buy tissues with lotion in them; I live on Puffs Plus® myself. And what you've heard about chicken soup is true. Research has shown that hot chicken soup really does break up congestion and clear the nasal passages!

## Sinusitis:

- Use OTC pain medicine for facial pain.
- Inhale steam for several minutes every few hours to loosen mucus.
- Choose symptom-specific OTC remedies; it is better to take two different pills that specifically treat your symptoms than one combination pill that contains medicine you don't need.
- Use nasal saltwater (saline) spray 4 to 6 times a day to help keep the membranes moist and promote drainage. To make your own saline nasal spray, add one-quarter teaspoon of table salt to 8 ounces of warm water. For extra safety, boil the tap water first and use it after it has cooled.
- Drink plenty of fluids to avoid dehydration and keep the mucus flowing; hot fluids (such as hot tea) may help increase mucus flow.
- Apply warm (moist if you like) compresses on the face to reduce discomfort. Or cold may work better. Choose what feels best to you.
- For allergic sinusitis, check with your HCP about prescription antihistamines or anti-inflammatory nasal sprays.

## Colds:

- Check with your HCP or pharmacist to choose the proper OTC medicine(s) to treat your symptoms.
- Sleep and drink plenty of fluids.
- Resist the urge to reach for a drug remedy first for a stuffy nose; instead, inhale steam, have some hot chicken soup, rest, and drink plenty of fluids.

■ Drink hot herbal tea at bedtime. This can clear your nose and help you sleep. Adding a spoonful of honey can provide a gentle sedative effect, so you can fall asleep before your nose plugs up again.

## Allergies:

■ Allergy treatment is very complex so work with your HCP.

■ Take antihistamines. They block the histamine that is responsible for most of the nasal congestion, itching, and symptoms. Nonsedating antihistamines are now available OTC, but they are expensive.

■ Avoid allergens if you can identify them.

## Nosebleed:

■ Pinch the nostrils closed and hold pressure for 15 minutes—by the clock—while you breathe through your mouth.

■ Apply a cold pack across the bridge of your nose, just above where your fingers are pinching it shut.

■ Sit slightly forward or in another comfortable upright position. Do *not* lie flat on our back or tilt your chin toward the ceiling, that position could make you choke on the blood.

■ Don't put anything like gauze or cotton balls in your nose to try to stop bleeding; they'll only need to be dug out later, and may rip off a scab.

■ Once the bleeding stops, don't blow your nose for at least 48 hours and don't pick your nose for at least a week.

## COLD REMEDIES

Decongestants are a big part of the multisymptom cold and flu market. They are often paired with antihistamines, and here's why: antihistamines make you drowsy, and decongestants can make you hyper. So the decongestants are used to offset the drowsiness caused by antihistamines. Check when a product touts a "nondrowsy" formula; chances are, you'll find a decongestant. Remedies that have day and night versions typically contain decongestants in the day version since they keep you awake and antihistamines (with or without the decongestant) in the night version to make you sleepy.

If you need a decongestant and an antihistamine, take both—for example, if you have a short-term seasonal allergy that completely plugs your nose in addition to your other allergy symptoms. But don't take medicine you don't need to fix side effects of another drug.

Decongestants work by constricting blood vessels. If mucous membranes are infected or irritated, they swell. Whenever blood vessels shrink, blood flow is reduced, and this reduces swelling. (It's the same reason you put ice on an injury; constrict the blood vessels and you'll have less swelling.) That's how decongestants open up your stuffy nose, by reducing the swelling in the membranes.

**Pseudoephedrine pills or liquid.**
Pseudoephedrine is the most common decongestant found in multisymptom remedies for colds, flu, allergies, and sinus trouble. Be sure to check the label for pseudephedrine, and think about whether you need to take a decongestant at all.

**Nasal sprays.**
Two leading ingredients in decongestant nasal sprays are oxymetazoline and phenylephrine hydrochloride. Again it is critical that you know if the nasal spray you are selecting is saltwater (saline) that will simply flush mucus out of your nose, or a decongestant that will shrink the blood vessels. If decongestant nasal sprays are used for more than two to three days, when they are stopped, the blood vessels will dilate, worsening congestion. This is called rebound. To avoid rebound, use decongestant nose sprays only for very short periods—three days, at most.

### ✚ When to consider

- If your nose is so stuffy you cannot breathe through it.
- If your ears get plugged up when you travel in an airplane, causing ear pain, a decongestant can open the Eustachian tubes that connect your middle ear with your throat, allowing the pressure to equalize and reducing the risk of pain.

### 🚫 Do not use

- If you have a history of heart disease or high blood pressure.
- If you are sensitive to substances that can increase your heart rate or blood pressure.
- If you have an overactive thyroid.
- If you have trouble urinating.

## ALLERGY REMEDIES

Antihistamines are drugs that block the histamine receptors in your body. When a substance you're allergic to enters your body, you respond by cranking up production of histamine. The histamine attaches to specialized cells called receptors, and bingo, you get the itching, burning eyes, runny nose, sneezing, and other symptoms that you're familiar with. If the histamine is released but the receptors are blocked, you either won't get those symptoms or they will be significantly less severe. Many antihistamines are available OTC, and within the past year, the first nonsedating antihistamine, loratadine, was switched from prescription only to OTC.

All of the OTC antihistamines except loratadine have drowsiness as a side effect. As a little experiment, take a walk down the sleep aids aisle in your local pharmacy. Most of the OTC medicines that will help you sleep use antihistamines to make you drowsy. (The ingredient diphenhydramine is particularly popular in OTC sleeping pills.) Next, look at the pain relievers that use "PM" on the label.

What's the difference between daytime medicines and PM medicines? Almost always, it's the addition of an antihistamine that will make you sleepy. Now that you know the secret, check labels carefully. If you have a headache at night, take a plain pain reliever, there's nothing magical about an OTC box that says PM on the label. You don't need to take an antihistamine if you don't have allergy symptoms. However, as an occasional OTC sleep aid, for example, when you're away from home, a medication such as Sominex can do the trick. The key is to know precisely what you are taking and why.

## ✚ When to consider

- To reduce allergy symptoms such as itching, hives, watery eyes, sneezing, or runny nose.
- To occasionally help you sleep.
- To treat motion sickness.

## 🚫 Do not use

Don't self-treat with an OTC antihistamine (check with your HCP first) if you:

- Have an enlarged prostate.
- Have glaucoma.
- Have trouble urinating.
- Are often constipated.
- Have any condition that causes dry eyes or particularly dry skin.

## LISTEN UP!

In today's instant-gratification world, it is hard to be a patient patient and let a cold, sinus infection, or allergy run its course. But in most cases, your nose knows what's best. As long as your sinuses can drain, time is your best ally.

# SORE THROAT

## NURSE'S NOTE

Sore throats generally fall into three categories: bacterial infections, viral infections, and irritation. Only bacterial infection should be treated with antibiotics. While we're in the neighborhood, we'll (ahem) talk about laryngitis, too.

Saying "Ahhhh" while someone looks in your throat is still one of the best ways to get the correct diagnosis!

## GET THEE TO THE ER

Sore throats rarely require an ER visit. The exceptions requiring a call to 911 are when:

■ Your throat hurts so badly that you are drooling because you can't swallow your own saliva.
■ Swelling in your throat is so great, it's hard for you to breathe, or when you breathe, you make squeaking noises.

## CALL YOUR HEALTH CARE PROVIDER

■ If you have a sore throat that lasts more than about 48 hours, and you don't have a cold or influenza.
■ If your sore throat comes with a fever.
■ If there are white patches or pus in the back of your throat (whether or not you still have tonsils).
■ If the glands in your neck are swollen or if opening your mouth or moving your jaw is very painful.
■ If you notice swollen glands in your armpits or groin in addition to those in your neck and have noticeable fatigue. (You could have mononucleosis.)
■ If you have laryngitis or are hoarse for no clear reason.
■ If changes in your voice last more than a week or two.

## COMMON CAUSES OF SORE THROAT

### Bacterial infection.

Fewer than half of all sore throats result from infection by any type of bacteria. A throat culture will make the diagnosis.

How you feel:
- Soreness in the throat comes on suddenly
- Really sick
- Feverish

Other indicators:
- Have few other symptoms
- May or may not know others who have been sick

Nurse's order:
- Take antibiotics from your HCP until they are all gone, even if you feel fine in a few days.
- Take OTC medication for pain and fever

### Viral infection.

Sore throats are common with viral illnesses such as colds and influenza. A sore throat caused by a viral infection can hurt just as much as one from a bacterial infection. In fact, in adults, sore throats that occur with mononucleosis can be so severe that it is hard to swallow, so people don't drink and get dehydrated. However, the degree of pain does not mean that you need antibiotics. Sore throats caused by a virus go away when the virus runs its course.

How you feel:
- Somewhat sick
- Soreness in the throat comes on gradually
- Body aches, headache
- Tired, without much energy

Other indicators:
- Low fever (if any)
- Know others who are sick

Nurse's order:
- Take OTC medications for pain

**Irritation.**
Many sore throats are caused by irritation from having allergies, being exposed to tobacco smoke, air pollution, inhaling other particulates, or breathing very dry air.

How you feel:
- Soreness in the throat
- Not sick or feverish

Other indicators:
- If allergy-related, will also have itchy, watery eyes; sneezing; and a runny nose
- Have been exposed to an allergen or irritant

**Laryngitis.**
Do you bark like a seal when you cough? When you try to talk, do only squeaks come out? Laryngitis, an inflammation of the vocal cords, can be due to either a viral infection (the same one that causes croup in kids) that's zeroed in on the vocal cords, or irritation from overuse, such as cheering loudly at a sporting event or trying to carry on a conversation in a noisy environment.

How you feel:
- Sick and fatigued, if caused by a virus
- Silly because you have an abnormal voice if you are not sick (if caused by overuse)

---

### ❓ Frequently Asked Questions

**Q.** *Is tonsillitis a bacterial or viral infection?*

**A.** A medical term ending in -itis usually means inflammation; tonsils can become inflamed from either a bacterial or viral infection.

**Q.** *What's the difference between croup and laryngitis?*

**A.** The main difference is the size of the airway. Infection with the virus that causes croup in a child will cause laryngitis in an adult. In both cases, the vocal cords swell. One millimeter of swelling in an adult is barely noticeable. In a child, that same swelling can reduce the size of his airway by one-quarter to one-half. What may be a simple nuisance for an adult can cause breathing trouble in a child.

Nurse's orders:
- Voice rest
- Drink plenty of fluids

## TECHNICALLY SPEAKING . . .

Two rare bacterial infections in the throat have the potential to cause serious breathing trouble. Epiglottitis is a bacterial infection of a structure called the epiglottis, which is the flapper valve that covers your airway so you can swallow without choking. If that valve becomes infected and swollen, it can block the airway instead of protecting it. An abscess in the back of the throat or around the tonsils can cause swelling so severe it nearly blocks the airway. Both of these are more common in children, but I have seen both in adults and they need immediate attention.

## NURSE'S WISDOM

- You may have a sore throat from breathing through your mouth because your nose is stuffed. Treat the nose and your throat will magically improve. When you can, consciously breathe through your nose. The inside of your nose warms and moistens the air, which protects your throat and vocal cords.

- Get a new toothbrush so you don't keep bringing germs into your mouth that can lead to another sore throat.
- Sucking on hard candy may make you more uncomfortable if it hurts to swallow, since the candy will make you swallow more often.
- Instead of trying to spray the back of your throat with an OTC numbing spray, try spraying it into a disposable cup and gargle with it instead. More medicine will get to the right place since your tongue won't be in the way.
- Be careful if you have used an inhaler for asthma. If you try to spray the medication into your mouth, you may reflexively take a deep breath at the same time and choke. You won't be in danger, but it will hurt.
- Regular OTC pain medicines will also treat sore throat.
- When you have laryngitis, whispering can be more irritating to your vocal cords than normal speech. Rest your voice as much as possible, but if you have to say something, just talk.
- Similarly, don't shout. If you do a lot of public speaking, use a microphone whenever you can and speak at a normal volume into the microphone to reduce voice strain.

## SELF-CARE

### Sore throat:
- Drink plenty of fluids—as much as you can.
- Eat popsicles and ice cream or any other cold delight that goes down smoothly and soothes the pain. They'll also stave off dehydration.
- Take an OTC pain reliever of choice on a regular schedule, following label instructions to reduce pain and fever, if present.
- Gargle with warm saltwater (1 teaspoon of salt in 8 ounces of water). Do not swallow. Gargle, swish, and spit.

- Increase the humidity in your home (at least 30%), particularly if it's winter and the heat is on.
- Don't smoke and stay away from irritants you can breathe in.

### Laryngitis:
- Shhhh. Don't talk.
- Don't smoke or expose yourself to smoke in the air.
- Drink plenty of fluids.
- Breathe in steam: put your head over a bowl of hot water; or close the bathroom door, turn the shower on hot, have a seat somewhere outside the shower, and breathe in the warm mist.

## SORE THROAT REMEDIES

Unfortunately, there isn't a magic prescription-strength throat remedy. If a potent local anesthetic could be sprayed into your throat by your HCP, you would be so numb you wouldn't be able to eat or drink because you might choke!

### Numbing/local anesthetic.
The most common ingredients in sore throat remedies are benzocaine, dyclonine, and phenol. These drugs will make your mouth and throat feel tingly and decrease your feeling of pain. However, you won't lose all sensation.

### Menthol.
This is a common ingredient in lozenges because it creates a cooling sensation in the throat that soothes the pain for many people.

## LISTEN UP!

It's easy to get dehydrated when you have a sore throat because it hurts to swallow. If you have a fever, the risk of dehydration is even greater. Think and drink. Popsicles and ice cream count toward your fluid intake, so knock yourself out! If you feel sore *and* guilty, sorbet and sherbet will do the trick, too.

## FEVER

### NURSE'S NOTE

Simply put, fever is a body temperature higher than normal. In otherwise healthy adults, a temperature above the traditional norm of 98.6 degrees Fahrenheit isn't considered a fever until you hit at least 100.5. Even if your "normal" temperature is lower than 98.6, you don't get fever credit until you're over 100.5, regardless of where you started. Experts today are less concerned about treating a fever just because it's an abnormal reading. In fact, many believe that fever is beneficial because when the body's temperature rises, it is less hospitable to viruses and bacteria. Fever may just be your ally in fighting infection. What this means is that you don't need to rush to treat a fever unless it is making you very uncomfortable, or if you have a preexisting health condition that you already know about from your HCP that a fever would worsen. The degree of fever is not as important as how you feel with the elevated temperature.

If you have a fever, but are able to go to work or school and can function (albeit at half speed), then you probably don't have something serious going on. People who are seriously ill with high fevers look sick, feel sick, and act sick. You can tell simply by looking at them there's something wrong.

### GET THEE TO THE ER

Head for the ER if you have a fever and:

- A severe headache and stiff neck, and regular room lighting hurts your eyes.

- Severe abdominal or back pain (with or without nausea or vomiting).
- A change in the level of consciousness, or the person with the fever is confused or hard to wake up.

## CALL YOUR HEALTH CARE PROVIDER

Call your HCP if you have any concerns about your fever or if:

- You develop a fever and a rash at the same time.
- The fever lasts more than three or four days.
- The fever is high—for example, more than 103 to 104 degrees Fahrenheit.
- Self-care does not reduce the fever at all.
- You have fevers that come and go and night sweats (awakening with wet hair at the nape of your neck, or damp PJs from perspiring).

## INSIDER INFO

Beware of ear thermometers! The initial research on these cool devices was done on unconscious patients immediately after open heart surgery. The ear temperature was compared with the blood temperature in and around the heart, and there was a good match. However, those carefully controlled conditions are very different from real life in which you buy a device at the drugstore, stick it in the ear, and push a button to get a reading.

A few years ago, traditional thermometers were set aside in favor of the new, timesaving technology. Now we know that an ear thermometer can miss a fever 25% to 35% of the time. Today, in health care settings, ear thermometers are generally used for screening. If it's very important to determine whether a patient has a fever, or to carefully monitor whether a fever is rising or falling, most HCPs will instead use the old reliable rectal temperature.

## COMMON SYMPTOMS OF FEVER

Fevers can make you feel hot or give you chills. You don't need to bundle up to "sweat it out," nor do you need to feel cold. Use common sense. Go to bed (or at least to the couch). Layer sheets and blankets so you can adjust the covers based on how warm or cold you feel. If you're hot, wear something lightweight; cotton is best to absorb perspiration. If you're cold, wear something comfy that will keep you from feeling chilled.

### Fever from a bacterial infection.

How you feel:
- Fine, then suddenly miserable in a short time, even a few hours
- One major symptom stands out, such as a sore throat, or abdominal pain, or a bad earache
- May or may not know other people who are sick

Nurse's order:
- Take antibiotics as prescribed by your HCP

### Fever from a viral infection.

How you feel:
- With the exception of influenza, a sickness that worsens gradually over a few days
- Achiness in the body and head
- Soreness in the throat
- Fatigued

Other indicators:
- Often know others who are sick, usually in the same household

Nurse's order:
- Take OTC medications for pain and fever
- Do not take antibiotics

## ? Frequently Asked Questions

**Q.** *Is it true that the higher the fever, the more serious the condition?*

**A.** Not necessarily. Younger people tend to get higher temperatures more easily from uncomplicated conditions like an ear infection, and older people may not have a fever even with a serious infection.

**Q.** *Do sponge baths and alcohol rubs reduce fever?*

**A.** Those methods were once common because they enhanced evaporation from the skin and thus lowered the body's temperature. But they can be uncomfortable and sometimes cause shivering. Experts now say not to use cold water or alcohol to lower a person's temperature. If you need to reduce a fever, start with OTC medicines. If you want to do something while waiting for the medicine to work, a warm—not hot—water bath is the best choice.

**Q.** *Is it true you're not supposed to use aspirin to treat an illness with a fever?*

**A.** That is true for children. A rare condition called Reye Syndrome can develop in some children with viral infections if they are treated with any drug from the aspirin family. For otherwise healthy adults, aspirin is a fine choice.

## TECHNICALLY SPEAKING . . .

Heat exhaustion and heat stroke can raise body temperature, but in this case it's not considered a fever. Heat exhaustion is essentially a severe form of dehydration (being properly hydrated helps regulate body temperature) when a person is overheated from being in a warm environment. Heat stroke occurs when the body loses the ability to regulate its temperature altogether. That's why medicines typically used to lower fevers won't have any effect on someone with a heat-related illness.

Fever, on the other hand, is the body's reaction to an infection or significant inflammation (such as rheumatoid arthritis).

## NURSE'S WISDOM

- To cool body temperature, place cold packs where large blood vessels are close to the skin surface—such as the armpits, folds of the groin, and the back of the neck—so that the blood you cool there will circulate around the body.
- Don't "starve a fever." Instead eat small, frequent meals to keep up with the increased metabolism that comes with a fever.
- Drink plenty of fluids to avoid dehydration, which can result from perspiring or not feeling like eating or drinking. Choose warm or cold beverages including water, fruit juices, or tea. Just make sure you drink. And if you're sleeping your way through the fever, have someone else in the household make sure you drink every time you wake up.
- Body temperature is always highest in the late afternoon and evening and lowest first thing in the morning.
- Be more aggressive about reducing fever if it's very hot outside and you don't have air conditioning. The fever combined with the hot environmental temperatures increases your risk for heat exhaustion.

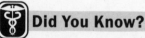 **Did You Know?**

Don't use ear thermometers while you're sitting in front of a fan, according to a University of Washington study. Nursing researchers compared ear and throat temperatures during whole body heating and cooling. When subjects' faces were cooled by a fan, their ear temperature decreased, but throat temperature (a more reliable indicator of body temperature) was unchanged. If you use an ear thermometer at home, be aware that a fan or cold cloth on the face could affect thermometer accuracy.

- Treating a fever is often more art than science; you can choose any of the OTC remedies you prefer.
- If you are treating a fever, take your temperature with a thermometer and check to see if your temperature is lower a few hours after taking one of the fever-reducing medicines. It doesn't make sense for you to take medicine if you can't (or don't) measure its effects. It's hard to know if a drug is working if you don't use a thermometer.
- If one type of medicine does not lower your temperature, try another. Some experts recommend alternating fever remedies—for example, a proper dose of acetaminophen, followed three hours later by a dose of ibuprofen, followed three hours later by acetaminophen, and so on. Others believe this only causes confusion and increases the risk of mistakes and overdose, but I've used this approach with success.

## SELF-CARE

Rest, drink plenty of fluids, and call your HCP if you're not improving in a few days. Take a fever-reducing drug such as acetaminophen, aspirin, or ibuprofen. Any questions? Call your HCP.

## FEVER REMEDIES

Three different types of drugs will reduce fever (they're all also pain relievers). Some experts recommend alternating categories of medicines for most effective relief.

### Acetaminophen.
Acetaminophen reduces fever by acting on the heat-regulating center of the brain.

### Aspirin.
Aspirin reduces fever by acting on the heat-regulating center of the brain; it reduces temperature by dilating small blood vessels in the skin.

## Ibuprofen and naproxen.

Ibuprofen and naproxen are nonsteroidal anti-inflammatory drugs (NSAIDs). These drugs interfere with prostaglandin synthesis, which produces chemical substances that cause inflammation and can also cause fever.

### ✚ When to consider

- To reduce a body temperature over 101 degrees Fahrenheit.
- When a fever is limiting your activities.

### 🚫 Do not use

- If you are sensitive to any of the ingredients in the treatments.
- If you consume three or more alcoholic beverages a day or if you have liver disease, check with your HCP before using any OTC fever-reducing medicine.
- If you are trying to reduce the body temperature of someone having heat exhaustion or heat stroke; they won't work.
- If you have a fever with other symptoms for which you are taking other OTC medicines. Exercise caution and read the label so as not to overdose on acetaminophen.
- More doses than recommended on the label.

## LISTEN UP!

If you have a fever and are not sick with an infection of some sort, see your HCP for a checkup. Read labels carefully when you choose an OTC treatment for your fever and the illness that goes along with it. Most multisymptom cold-flu-sinus preparations contain one of the three drugs used to reduce fever. To avoid an unintentional overdose, don't take separate fever medicine if acetaminophen, aspirin, or ibuprofen is already in the remedy you've selected. Also do not take more than the recommended dose of any fever-reducing OTC medicine.

# ■ STOMACH ACHES ■

## HEARTBURN

### NURSE'S NOTE

Antacids are one of the top-selling OTC remedies in the United States, and since a new type of heartburn pill switched from prescription to OTC in the fall of 2003, no doubt the money we spend on these drugs will rise.

Stomach remedies for self-treatment of heartburn should be used occasionally, *not* every day unless your HCP says otherwise. If you have regular, frequent, or continuous symptoms, you need a checkup.

### GET THEE TO THE ER

Call 911 for a ride to the ER if:

- You have pain in your chest and are not sure what's causing it. Don't assume it is simple heartburn.
- If your "usual" heartburn sensation is different.
- If you have heartburn regularly and you vomit blood or dark brown material resembling coffee grounds.

■ If your heartburn occurs with severe abdominal pain or chest pain, or you are short of breath or lightheaded.

## CALL YOUR HEALTH CARE PROVIDER

■ If you have acid indigestion, heartburn, sour stomach, bloating, or gas more than once or twice a week.
■ If your symptoms are not easily related to a particular food.
■ If you have taken a remedy for two weeks and still have symptoms.

## COMMON CAUSE OF HEARTBURN

When you eat, your stomach produces more acid to digest the food. The food fills the stomach and puts more pressure on the opening back to the esophagus. Sometimes the acid flows backward from the stomach into the esophagus, causing pain. The technical term for this is reflux. (see page 98 if you have a cough associated with your reflux pain.)

How you feel:
■ Burning sensation or pain in chest
■ Burning sensation or pain is worse when lying down, or after a meal
■ Burning sensation or pain is not affected by movement or breathing
■ Burning in throat, or an acid or sour taste in throat and mouth especially after a burp

Other indicators:
■ Discomfort worsens when you recline in an easy chair or lie down after eating

Nurse's orders:
■ Take OTC antacids for occasional symptoms

## Frequently Asked Questions

Q. *How do I know whether to take an antacid, a liquid, chewable tablets, or some sort of acid blocker before I eat or after?*

A. I wish there were a simple answer, but there isn't. If you have the occasional sour stomach or heartburn, I'd recommend a liquid antacid when you're home, and a chewable if you're out and about and need something portable like Tums. Or if the "pink stuff" works for you, use it. If you check to make sure you have antacid whenever you leave home because you have frequent symptoms, that's a sign you need to see your HCP. Hold off on the acid blockers (keep reading to learn about them) until you've had a talk with your HCP and get a recommendation to use one or another of them for your particular situation. You may want to check out Gaviscon chewable tablets that can reduce reflux episodes by creating a foam barrier on top of the stomach acid. If there's backwash, it will be the foam, not the acid that enters the esophagus.

■ Contact your HCP if your symptoms require an OTC stomach remedy for more than two weeks

## NURSE'S WISDOM

■ Chew antacid chewable tablets completely before swallowing, they will work faster if the medicine is in tiny pieces in your stomach.

■ These medicines are effective for occasional use to treat a sour stomach when you've had one too many tacos, or that sauce had a lot more garlic than you expected.

■ Some of these are calcium based and Tums is approved as a calcium supplement.

■ Antacids that coat the stomach and neutralize acid can block absorption of other drugs taken at the same time.

■ Some antacids cause constipation or diarrhea.

■ There are now three different types of heartburn remedies
OTC; the choice of treatment for recurring symptoms is not a
simple one. Sometimes, an examination with a lighted instrument passed through the mouth and into the stomach is required to confirm what condition is causing symptoms (see
page 294), thus making it even more challenging for consumers to make an intelligent choice in the pharmacy aisle
based on symptoms alone.

■ There's a lot of money to be made in this OTC market seg-
ment; do not let commercials help you make your own diagnosis. You can get useful information from commercials that
you can then discuss with your HCP or pharmacist to come to
the right choice for you based on your condition and any other
medicines you may be taking.

## SELF-CARE

■ Eat smaller, more frequent meals (but don't increase your
caloric intake).

■ Stay away from carbonated beverages that increase air in your
stomach.

■ Cut down on alcohol, and uncoated aspirin and anti-
inflammatory pills that can cause stomach irritation.

■ Don't eat within two to three hours of going to bed for the
night.

■ Stop smoking. Smoking increases stomach acid (see smoking
cessation, page 104).

■ Maintain a healthy weight, and don't wear clothing that is
tight around the waist.

## HEARTBURN REMEDIES

### Antacids.
These medicines neutralize acid in the stomach. Most contain either
aluminum (not as common), calcium, or magnesium; some are a

combination of these ingredients. Sodium bicarbonate is commonly in fizzy tablets that dissolve in water, and can increase blood pressure in sensitive people. Bismuth subsalicylate—the "pink stuff"—coats the stomach lining and is a weak acid neutralizer.

### Acid blockers.

Instead of neutralizing what's already in the stomach, these medicines decrease the amount of acid produced. One way is by blocking receptor cells that, when stimulated, increase acid secretion; the other is to block the final step of acid production. Drugs that block the receptor cells are cimetidine, famotidine, nizatidine, and ranitidine. The drug that blocks the final step of acid production is omeprazole.

### Anti-gas.

Simethicone reduces the surface tension of bubbles, which is thought to disperse air more evenly through the stomach and intestine. Experts disagree on the efficacy of this drug.

### LISTEN UP!

Far too many people ignore the label warnings and take OTC heartburn medicines for a long time without a visit to the HCP for a diagnosis. In the long term, this can be dangerous if a serious condition goes untreated!

# DIARRHEA AND CONSTIPATION

### NURSE'S NOTE

Millions of people have abnormal bowel function. Sometimes, it is due to a short-term bug, irritation, or medication side effect; in other cases, the abnormal function is a chronic condition. It's important not to go overboard in an effort to have "perfectly normal" function; if you regularly take OTC remedies, overtreatment of diarrhea can cause constipation, and overtreatment of constipation can cause diarrhea.

The key to successful management of long-term abnormal bowel function is individualized care. For irritable bowel syndrome, the best approach is trial and error. For example, some people may find oatmeal helps maintain regularity; in others, it may cause diarrhea or constipation. The challenge is to throw the book (not this one, of course!) out the window, and listen to your body. If a particular food causes problems, remove it from your diet and move on. With patience, you will have a very good sense of what foods help your intestines work best and which to avoid.

## GET THEE TO THE ER

- If there is significant body fluid loss through diarrhea and vomiting prevents fluid replacement by drinking, it's better to get to the ER earlier rather than later for treatment of dehydration.
- If diarrhea has bright red blood, or a black, tar-like appearance.

## CALL YOUR HEALTH CARE PROVIDER

- If your bowel function is abnormal for more than a few weeks without an obvious cause.
- If diarrhea has some blood in it; if you don't get through to your HCP right away, go to the ER.
- If you need to ask about using an OTC diarrhea remedy, when you should use it, and which one to use.
- If diarrhea or constipation begins after starting a new medicine.
- If you have frequent bouts of diarrhea with no identifiable cause.

- If you are taking a constipation remedy more than once a week.
- If you have diarrhea and vomiting, but are not yet dehydrated.
- If you have not produced any urine in eight hours; lack of urine indicates significant dehydration.
- If you have a fever with diarrhea or severe abdominal pain (not just cramps).

## COMMON SYMPTOMS OF DIARRHEA AND CONSTIPATION

### Diarrhea.

Diarrhea consists of watery, loose, nonformed bowel movements. It occurs when the intestinal contents move through the system so quickly that water is not reabsorbed back into the body. When you have diarrhea, the first focus should be on increasing fluid intake to avoid dehydration. There is debate even among specialists about when to treat diarrhea and when to let it run its course. Diarrhea usually occurs when there is some type of infection or irritation in the intestine, and the body needs to get rid of it. See if you can hang on for 24 hours before reaching for a remedy. Be sure to drink plenty of fluids.

How you feel:
- Like you have to go—*right now*
- May have abdominal cramping

Other indicators:
- Your bowel movements are more watery than solid
- You may be moving your bowels three or four times per hour

Nurses's orders:
- Maintain fluid intake to minimize risk of dehydration

### Constipation.

This is a condition in which bowel movements occur three times a week or less. With constipation, fecal material is hard and dry, usually from being in the intestine so long that all moisture has been absorbed back into the body.

Nurse's orders:
If you don't have a complicating medical condition:

■ Increase fluid intake
■ Increase activity, such as walking for exercise
■ Increase bulk or fiber in your diet

If you get in the habit of using a laxative daily "to stay regular," the muscles in your intestine will slow down and not function properly without a laxative. You can get "hooked," so proceed with caution.

Note that constipation alone is not a reason to go to the ER; if stools are changing, follow up with your HCP.

How you feel:
■ Bowel movements are infrequent (fewer than three times per week) and food intake is not significantly reduced
■ Fecal material is very hard, often in small amounts (rabbit pellets)
■ It is difficult to pass the stool; sometimes it feels like the rectum is still full even after a movement
■ There is a significant change in habits to less frequent, smaller, and harder stools

## TECHNICALLY SPEAKING ...

Two long-term conditions can cause either constipation or diarrhea, or alternating bouts of both: inflammatory bowel disease and irritable bowel syndrome. Irritable bowel syndrome (IBS) is a disorder of intestinal function. The pattern of symptoms varies from person to person, but is typically characterized by either predominantly diarrhea or predominantly constipation, and excessive gas that causes bloating and abdominal pain because the intestine is distended. Normally, the intestinal muscles move in a consistent wave-like motion, which pushes the solid waste through the bowel, ideally reaching a point in which enough water is reabsorbed so that the stool is in solid form, but it is expelled before it dries out and becomes hard. In IBS, the muscles push material through too quickly or too slowly.

## ? Frequently Asked Questions

Q. Why can't I just use antidiarrhea medicine right away?

A. Antidiarrhea medicines slow bowel function down. If a toxin is present from an infection, you don't want to trap it with OTC remedies. The diarrhea is the body's way to eliminate the toxin. That's why it's a good idea to check in with your HCP and describe the pattern of your symptoms and get advice for a particular illness.

Q. Sometimes I get diarrhea when I am nervous. Should I treat that?

A. That's normal—part of the fight-or-flight reflex that occurs when your body produces adrenalin. If you get nervous before you need to make a business presentation, for example, you could try a loperamide pill beforehand so you're not interrupted during your talk.

Q. My friends use laxatives to lose weight if they eat too much. What's wrong with that?

A. Taking laxatives in order to have diarrhea to lose weight causes two problems: One, if you do it often enough, your intestine won't remember how to work properly and you'll have to take drugs in order to have a normal pattern. Two, if you have diarrhea, you will lose substances from the body called electrolytes. Electrolytes are particles essential to muscle functioning, particularly proper heart function. If you lose potassium and sodium by forcing your body to have diarrhea, you could have dangerous abnormal heart rhythms. People have died from abusing laxatives in this way.

**Did You Know?**

Nursing researchers evaluated 97 women with IBS to see if changes in bowel pattern were related to psychological distress. Forty percent of women showed a positive correlation between daily psychological distress and daily gastrointestinal symptoms. Psychological distress can be an important component in IBS symptom experience (whether as a cause or as a result) and thus should be considered when you and your health care provider are designing treatment strategies. Don't focus only on the intestine—think about the body-mind connection as well.

Some people never have "normal" function, while others have bouts of abnormal function. The cause has not been pinned down. IBS does not lead to serious complications.

Inflammatory bowel disease (IBD), on the other hand, is a group of disorders in which the lining of the intestine becomes inflamed. The two most well-known illnesses are Crohn's disease and ulcerative colitis. Diarrhea and weight loss predominate, stools can be bloody, and abdominal pain can be severe. Accumulation of scar tissue can require surgery to relieve blockage of the intestine. People with IBD may have a higher risk of colon cancer because the cells lining the intestine are chronically irritated, which can lead to abnormal cell growth.

## NURSE'S WISDOM

- Some people are particularly sensitive to lactose in dairy products; see if you notice a connection between dairy consumption, such as an ice cream sundae, and subsequent diarrhea.
- Overuse of antacids containing magnesium can cause diarrhea—remember, milk of magnesia is a laxative.
- Diarrhea can be contagious; microbes can be spread, particularly if the stool is pure water and splashes. Wash your hands

frequently, and do not prepare food for other members of the household until the illness has passed.

■ If you have diarrhea without nausea or vomiting, you can be a little more patient about treating the diarrhea because you can replace the fluids you're losing by drinking.

■ Be aware that thickening agents in liquid form can bind to other medicines. Do not take these OTC antidiarrhea medicines with other medicines.

■ If you have both vomiting and diarrhea, dehydration is a real danger. The thickening agent that is not absorbed into the body may be your best first choice to get the diarrhea under control and reduce the fluid loss from the intestine. The challenge can be the taste of the two remedies; bismuth subsalicylate and kaolin with pectin can be strong if you are nauseated to begin with.

■ Be aware that bismuth subsalicylate—the "pink stuff"—has an aspirin-like base; do not use it if you have an aspirin allergy or sensitivity.

■ Don't be timid about dosing once you decide to use one of these remedies; particularly with the thickening agents, underdosing is common. Follow the instructions on the label to take a dose after each loose bowel movement.

■ If you are selecting a constipation remedy, don't be confused by packages that say things like "constipation relief made for a woman." These drugs don't know and don't care whether they are working on a male or female intestine.

■ Some people are very sensitive to these drugs, so if you buy one of these medicines, start with the smallest package and see how you respond.

■ Choose a single-ingredient product so if you get bad cramps or other side effects, you'll know what particular drug caused your problem.

■ Be aware that many constipation remedies are full of sugar and salt—important to note if you are on a restricted diet. Read labels carefully.

## SELF-CARE

### Diarrhea (short term):

- Do not stress your system with solid food if diarrhea is a short-term problem; stick with liquids for the first 12 to 24 hours.
- Drink plenty of fluid to balance the losses. Don't forget that salt helps you retain fluid, so during this period of potential dehydration, choose fluids such as chicken bouillon since it has more salt than plain chicken broth.
- After resting the intestine, introduce solids that will add bulk such as rice and bananas.
- Stay away from alcohol and any other potentially irritating foods and drinks.

### Constipation (short term):

- Constipation commonly occurs in busy people who don't have time to go to the bathroom when they get a signal, to exercise regularly, to drink plenty of fluids, and to plan what to eat and when. The first element of self-care is to do simple things: as soon as you feel the urge to move your bowels, go to the bathroom; increase your fluid intake; cut out the food on the run; and exercise.
- If these measures don't do the trick, try a bulk supplement such as methylcellulose or psyllium powder, well dissolved in at least 8 ounces of water daily.
- If you have hemorrhoids or anal pain or a fissure that causes pain, making you avoid moving your bowels, see your HCP for diagnosis and treatment so you can get back to normal.

## DIARRHEA REMEDIES

There are two approaches to treating diarrhea: one is to thicken the stool, the other is to relieve spasms of the intestinal muscles.

### Thickeners.

Attapulgite and kaolin with pectin absorb water, bacteria, and toxins from within the intestine and allow them to pass through the bowel in a more solid form. They are not absorbed into the body in any way and are much less likely to result in constipation.

## Spasm reliever.
Loperamide blocks the nerve signals to the intestine's muscles, slowing the spasms that cause frequent bowel movements.

## Combination drug.
Bismuth subsalicylate ("pink stuff") stimulates the body to absorb fluids from the intestines, binds with or neutralizes toxins of some bacteria, and decreases the irritation of the intestinal lining.

## ✚ When to consider

- If you've had diarrhea for more than 24 hours.
- If you feel dehydrated, are thirsty all the time, weak, and a little lightheaded when you stand.
- If you are not vomiting.

## 🚫 Do not use

- For the first 24 hours if possible.
- If you are passing blood.
- If you are having alternating episodes of diarrhea and constipation, unless directed by your HCP.

## CONSTIPATION REMEDIES

There are two classifications for constipation remedies: stool softener or laxative. There is only one stool softener, but there are four types of laxatives. Because long-term use can disturb normal bowel function, you should turn to these only when absolutely necessary.

**Stool softener.**
Docusate is a detergent that helps pull water into the formed stool to soften the mass. The presence of softer, more bulky stool in the intestine gently stimulates muscle contractions to move the stool out of the body.

**Laxative—bulk-forming.**
Bran, psyllium, and methylcellulose are forms of fiber that are not digested before passing into the intestine. There, they increase the bulk of the stool, and as with stool softeners, the increased bulk helps Mother Nature move the stool through the intestine more effectively. These remedies are gentle and are probably most similar to the natural function you could stimulate by consuming more fiber in your diet and drinking lots of water. If you choose this remedy, by sure you drink lots of fluids to reduce any risk of the fiber clumping together and causing a blockage. Make sure the powder form is completely dissolved before you drink it down, and know that these remedies can cause gas and bloating in sensitive people, so start slowly.

**Laxative—osmotic.**
These remedies include glycerin suppositories, magnesium citrate, magnesium hydroxide (milk of magnesia), and sodium phosphate (often in enema form). They work by pulling water into the intestine. The increased water softens and bulks up the stool. This bulk stretches the intestinal walls, causing the muscles to contract and move the now softer stool toward the rectum. These remedies tend to work more abruptly than other types of laxatives, so you don't want to use one just before you leave home for the day. You'll usually have a movement in 30 minutes to 3 hours. These drugs are often used to empty the intestines for surgery or tests (see bowel prep, p. 289). In sensitive people, these laxatives can cause significant cramping. You may want to chill liquid forms of these medicines to kill the taste.

**Laxative—stimulant.**
The most common, bisacodyl and senna, work by directly stimulating the muscles in the walls of the large intestine, moving the stool

forward. These laxatives are most likely to cause cramping, particularly if the stool is hard and dry and difficult to move. Note that the once-popular ingredient phenolphthalein was reclassified as "not generally safe and effective" by the FDA in 1999. Stimulant laxatives of this type are most likely to be habit forming, and can cause "lazy bowel syndrome" in which the intestine requires the stimulus of the drug so that the muscles will contract.

**Laxative—lubricant.**
Mineral oil and castor oil lead the way here; they coat the stool so there is less resistance to movement through the intestine. These lubricants shouldn't be your first choice for a few reasons: they interfere with the body's absorption of vitamins A, D, E, and K; the oil can leak from the rectum; and if the oil gets breathed in as you swallow, serious lung irritation can result.

## ✚ When to consider

- If you have been ill and your physical activity has been significantly reduced.
- If you have not had success by increasing the fiber in your diet, the amount of water you drink, and your physical activity.
- When you are taking medicines recommended or prescribed by your HCP, and the medicines (commonly opioid pain medicine and some high blood pressure medicines) cause a temporary bout of constipation.
- On the advice of your HCP.

## 🚫 Do not use

- If you have severe abdominal pain associated with a sudden change in bowel habits.
- If you have nausea and vomiting.
- If you have rectal bleeding and don't know why.

## LISTEN UP!

There is no rule that states you must have a bowel movement every day. "Normal" can range from two to three movements a day to three movements per week. Constipation can be managed in many ways without laxatives, and no laxative is completely risk free. Constipation remedies should be a last resort, not a first choice.

You may have food poisoning if you suddenly develop nausea, vomiting, and constipation, and if you know other people who are similarly ill who ate the same food you did—often at a picnic or other event. If you don't have a fever or bloody diarrhea, you can self-treat as long as you're not dehydrated.

# ABDOMINAL PAIN

## NURSE'S NOTE

There's good and bad news about a stomach ache, more formally called abdominal pain. The good news is that it's rarely serious and seldom requires surgery. The bad news is that it's very common. Abdominal pain is a challenge to HCPs because it's so subjective; a sensation that one person may notice but not worry about unless it worsens will cause others to call 911, convinced they have appendicitis. In this section, I'll explain the clues that help separate serious conditions from those that are run of the mill.

## GET THEE TO THE ER

Your belly ache earns you an ambulance ride to the ER if:

- You have severe pain that prevents you from sleeping or doing much of anything for more than four hours.
- You have severe pain and are vomiting.

- You have severe pain and your temperature is 101 degrees Fahrenheit or higher.
- You have severe pain and you feel faint.
- You have severe pain and know (or suspect) you are pregnant.
- Your abdominal muscles are rigid, like a board (and you don't have abs to die for).
- You have bright red bloody diarrhea or dark stools resembling tar.
- You are vomiting blood.
- You have pain with both vomiting and diarrhea and are severely dehydrated.

## CALL YOUR HEALTH CARE PROVIDER

- If pain is bad enough that you'd stay home from work, for example, but not so severe you're going straight to the ER.
- If the pain comes and goes in a predictable pattern.
- If pain is related to meals in some way.
- If pain is related to consuming particular foods or beverages.
- If you have pain, notice an increase in gas, and are bloated—particularly if the bloating is significant enough to make your clothes (particularly pants) too tight to wear.
- If you have continuous pain lasting more than three days.

## INSIDER INFO

If your pain is such that someone else is reading this for you while you're yelling, "I don't care where we go, just get rid of this pain!!!!," then go to the closest ER. If you are reading this and pondering your options, a call to the HCP who knows you best is a good place to start. For women, it may be tricky figuring out whether to call the primary care provider or the gynecologist.

How your abdominal pain gets evaluated is largely determined by where you go for treatment. Your primary HCP will usually have to do less of a work-up because he or she knows your medical history and hopefully whether you are a worrier or a minimizer.

At the other end of the spectrum is the teaching hospital ER, where every patient with abdominal pain must have their rectal temperature taken and receive a digital rectal exam. If you are female and between 16 and 60 years of age, they'll throw in a pelvic exam for good measure to make sure they've explored all the possible causes for your pain. (Also, a rule of ER practice is: "A woman is pregnant unless proven otherwise.")

Another key aspect of evaluating abdominal pain is the degree of inflammation of the abdominal wall's lining. The inflammation, called peritonitis (PAIR-uh-ten-EYE-tiss), is hard to miss; pain spikes when there is abdominal wall motion, such as from a cough or going over bumps in a car or ambulance. Be sure to mention if you're feeling this.

Pain severity is a key factor in diagnosing abdominal pain, but people have different pain tolerance. Here are the questions you'll be asked, so if you're not in agony, you can think about them in advance.

- Is the pain so bad that it prevents you from going to work or school, or from getting off the couch or out of bed? Or are you able to function despite having pain?
- Where is the pain? Can you point to the pain precisely with one finger, or is the pain in a more general area, closer to the size of your palm? Is the pain more intense in one place but shoots or seems to move to a second, separate location? Or is it only in one area?
- Can you pinpoint the exact moment the pain started, or has it crept up gradually? What were you doing when the pain started? Try to remember what you ate; whether you were injured, fell, or were in an accident; if you were under a lot of stress; if you had an operation; if you started new medicine— prescription, OTC, herbal, nutritional supplement; or if there is anything else you can think of that might be related to the start of the pain.
- Is the pain you have now the same as when it first started, or

has it changed? For example, did it start as an ache and become a stabbing pain? Has the pain been continuous since it started, or does it come and go? Sudden, severe pain is usually continuous. Unless you have pain every minute of every day, it's not considered continuous.

■ Have you had a similar pain before (whether you sought care or not)? You may forget unless you think carefully about it. People with gallstones, for example, may have episodes of pain many months apart, and they often don't realize the episodes are related. If you have pain that comes and goes, does it start out mild, get bad, and then fade away, or do you feel fine, then wham, you're in pain?

■ Have you noticed certain things that make the pain better or worse? How about eating (particular foods or drinks), moving your bowels (or not), taking medicines (or not), moving in a certain position (flexing your hips, standing up straight, lying in a fetal position), or doing certain things (having sexual intercourse, walking down stairs, pressing on the brake when you're driving)?

## COMMON CAUSES OF SHORT-TERM ABDOMINAL PAIN

### Appendicitis.
The appendix has no known function; appendicitis occurs when the appendix becomes inflamed and infected. Appendicitis is the most common cause for urgent abdominal surgery (and is the condition that most people who come to the ER with abdominal pain worry about).

How you feel:
■ Pain begins as general pain around the navel, and within four to six hours, becomes severe and moves to lower right abdomen
■ Pain around the navel that gets worse over four to six hours but does not move to lower right abdomen

■ Pain much worse with any movement, especially when coughing or going over bumps in the car on the way to get medical care

Other indicators:
■ May have nausea or vomiting
■ May have low fever

Nurse's order:
■ Have surgery to remove the inflamed appendix

## Gastroenteritis.

This inflammation of the stomach and intestines is most commonly caused by viral infection or food poisoning.

How you feel:
■ Sudden, cramping pain in the abdomen
■ Pain not usually severe but can worsen in "waves"
■ Significantly nauseated with vomiting and diarrhea
■ Pain doesn't increase with movement
■ Low fever
■ Dehydration, which can result from severe vomiting and diarrhea

Nurse's order:
■ If you can keep fluids down, choose clear liquids such as salty chicken bouillon or apple juice
■ Check in with your HCP about whether to take OTC medicine to stop the diarrhea

## Bladder infection.

This is more common in women than men because the tube leaving the bladder is so much shorter. Anyone who has had a bladder infection will recognize another one.

How you feel:
■ Severe pain or burning while urinating

- Sensation of needing to urinate often
- Cramping pain in lower central abdomen from bladder spasms

Other indicators:
- Cloudy or bloody urine (blood comes from irritation of the bladder lining and is scary, but not serious)
- Passing of only small amounts of urine

Nurse's orders:
- Provide a urine specimen that can be examined and cultured to identify bacteria.
- Take antibiotics prescribed by your HCP until they are all gone regardless of how soon you feel better.

## COMMON CAUSES OF LONG-TERM ABDOMINAL PAIN OR ABDOMINAL PAIN THAT COMES AND GOES

### Diverticulitis.
A diverticulum (dye-ver-TIC-you-lum) is a little pouch that forms in the wall of the large intestine. If you develop these pouches, you have diverticulosis. When one or more of the pouches become inflamed or infected, it's called diverticulitis.

How you feel:
- Crampy pain that is worse in left lower abdomen
- Pain may spike when you cough or if area is pressed
- Pain may occur after eating undigestible foods such as nuts, popcorn, or seeds
- Pain often decreases after bowel movement
- May be nauseated
- Feverish

Nurse's order:
- Limit your diet to rest intestines
- Take antibiotics as prescribed if infection is present

**Gallbladder disease.**
The gallbladder stores bile, which aids in fat digestion. Pain occurs when the gallbladder becomes inflamed; 90% of the time, this happens when gallstones block the opening through which bile flows. Gallstones are present in about 1 to 6 people in every 1,000. They're usually not treated unless they cause symptoms, which happens about 20% of the time.

How you feel:
- Sharp pain just below the right rib cage; pain may extend to back or right shoulder
- Pain often episodic (in "attacks")—often after eating fatty foods
- Pain may spike if abdomen is pressed, especially under the ribs
- Nauseated with or without vomiting
- May be feverish

Nurse's order:
- Don't eat or drink until pain subsides
- Consider surgery, but note that the surgeon will not perform surgery until you are symptom free

**Gas.**
The normal digestive process produces gas. Sometimes gas is released through the stomach, as a burp; it can also be released through the anus, called, um, in polite company, flatulence. Trapped gas can stretch the intestine, causing pain. Your belly may look bloated, too, and clothes may be tight.

How you feel:
- Pain that may feel like continuous tenderness, or may consist of occasional sharp pain
- Tenderness all over the abdomen when touched

Other indicators:
- Symptoms worse after eating high fiber foods, particularly beans

- No fever, nausea, or vomiting
- No change in bowel habits

Nurse's order:
- Take OTC medications that reduce gas in the intestine (many experts say they don't work, but if they do the trick for you, stick with them)
- Take OTC dietary enzymes, such as Beano, which prevent gas production
- Change your diet to avoid foods that cause excess gas

### Gastritis or ulcer.

Gastritis is an inflammation of the stomach lining. An ulcer is a crater formed when there is a break in the stomach's protective lining (gastric ulcer) or the lining of first part of the small intestine, as the intestine leaves the stomach (duodenal [doo-ODD-uh-null] ulcer). We used to think duodenal ulcers were caused by excess acid; now we know they are actually caused by a bacterial infection called *H. pylori*. Gastritis can be caused by the same bacteria and from irritants such as foods, medicines, and alcoholic beverages. Nonsteroidal anti-inflammatory drugs are one of the most common culprits. Eating may relieve pain or burning in the upper abdomen.

How you feel:
- Pain or burning in the upper abdomen
- Pain that gets worse after drinking heavily, taking anti-inflammatory medications, or being under stress
- Pain does not get worse when you move around or are examined
- Maybe nauseated, but vomiting not common

Other indicators:
- No fever
- No change in bowel patterns

---

**? Frequently Asked Questions**

Q. *Is it more serious if pain starts after vomiting?*

A. Actually, just the opposite is true. Pain followed by vomiting is more likely when there's a condition that will require surgery.

---

Nurse's order:

- Reduce stomach irritants (particularly OTC medicines and alcohol)
- Take acid-reducing medications (OTC or prescription)
- Have your HCP test for bacteria

## NURSE'S WISDOM

- Don't self-treat abdominal pain with an enema or laxative unless you are certain what the problem is.
- Heat therapy can reduce the pain from bladder spasm; air-activated single-use instant heat pads (originally designed for menstrual cramps) applied over the lower abdomen are ideal.
- During a bladder infection, limit drinking caffeine and alcohol, which can irritate the lower urinary tract and stimulate urination, which is already painful enough.
- Most bladder infections are from bacteria normally in the intestine. Women should *not* use toilet tissue in a wiping motion from back to front as this can transfer bacteria from the anus to the urethra (the tube through which urine leaves the bladder); bacteria can move up the urethra and into the bladder.
- Women prone to bladder infections should limit exposure to potential external irritants, such as colored toilet tissue that contains dye, bubble bath, douche, and perfumed cleansers.
- Sexually active women should urinate before and after sexual intercourse, and discuss their options for birth control with

their HCP; diaphragms can slightly increase risk for women already prone to bladder infections.

■ Women taking antibiotics to treat a bladder infection often get a vaginal yeast infection because the antibiotics kill off the normal bacteria that keep the yeast in check. Taking supplements such as acidophilus and eating yogurt with active bacterial cultures can help reduce the risk.

■ You can reduce the risk of diverticulosis flare-ups by eating a high-fiber diet; if you're not consuming much fiber, increase the amount slowly over a few weeks to give your digestive system a chance to adjust.

■ If intestinal gas is a problem, try eliminating dairy products from your diet and see if you notice a difference. If gas is noticeably reduced, reintroduce them slowly and monitor your response.

## SELF-CARE

### Bladder infection:

■ If you are not sure if you have a bladder infection, you can test your urine at home with AZO Test Strips. The strips contain pads that change color if white blood cells or bacterial by-products are present in the urine.

■ OTC phenazopyridine reduces urinary pain. Use *while waiting* to see your HCP, *not instead of* seeing your HCP; delaying care can allow the infection to spread to the kidney, which becomes a much more serious condition.

■ Drink cranberry juice to increase acidity of urine.

■ Drink 10 to 15 8-ounce glasses of fluid per day to flush the urinary system.

■ Take an OTC pain reliever of your choice.

### Diverticulitis:

■ If you're having an attack, get immediate medical care.

## Gallbladder disease:

■ If you're having an attack, get immediate medical care.

## Gas:

■ Try OTC remedies containing simethicone, which can reduce gas (even though experts disagree about this).

■ Drink hot liquids, particularly mint or chamomile tea, which provide relief for some people.

■ To reduce gas pain, lie on your back and pull your knees to your chest; this will help the air to move through the intestines, so you can expel the gas.

■ Taking a walk after meals can help air and solids move through the intestine.

## Gastritis or ulcer:

■ Use OTC acid reducers *until* you see your HCP, *not instead of* seeing your HCP.

■ If antibiotics are prescribed, take all pills exactly as directed. It's a multidrug regimen and can be a bit complicated, so be sure you understand what you need to do.

■ Reduce irritants such as plain (choose coated aspirin such as Ecotrin instead) aspirin, anti-inflammatory drugs, alcoholic beverages, and foods you find particularly troublesome (although a bland diet is not necessary).

■ Stop smoking and manage stress, which both increase stomach acid production.

## LISTEN UP!

Sudden, severe abdominal pain needs to be checked out right away in the ER. If you are going to the ER or have an urgent visit scheduled with your HCP to check out abdominal pain, don't eat or drink until an HCP clears you to do so. If you're with someone who's sick, make sure he doesn't eat or drink. Food or fluid consumption can make it more difficult to evaluate an abdominal condition, and if on the rare chance surgery is needed, it's better to have an empty stomach.

You can test for pregnancy and urine infections at home, but if those home results don't match your symptoms, forget the home test and see your HCP.

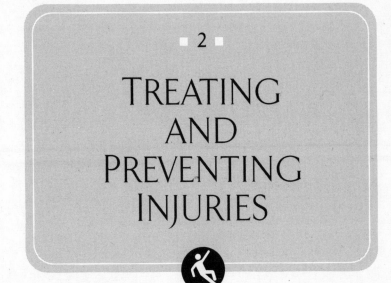

# 2

# TREATING AND PREVENTING INJURIES

# BITES AND STINGS

## NURSE'S NOTE

Stinging insects can transform an afternoon of summer fun to tears and fears as children and adults alike try to avoid the dreaded stings. For some people, stings hurt for a little while and go away; but for others, the sting of an insect can cause an allergic reaction that can be life-threatening.

There are four types of stinging insects: bees, yellow jackets, wasps, and hornets. Bees are the only insects that leave their stinger behind; thus, they can only sting once. Other insects can sting more than once if they are trapped in clothing or inside a sandal, for example.

## GET THEE TO THE ER

If a person has any of these signs or symptoms after a sting, call 911:

- Swelling of the face, particularly the lips, tongue, or eyelids
- Hives all over the body, particularly on the palms of the hands and the trunk
- Trouble breathing, chest tightness, coughing, or wheezing

- Dizziness, feeling lightheaded, or passing out
- Vomiting or diarrhea

## CALL YOUR HEALTH CARE PROVIDER

- If the area around the bite or sting turns red, if the red area gets larger, becomes warm to touch, or if red streaks lead away from the site and toward the body. All can be signs of infection.

Stinging insects are drawn to flowers where they collect pollen. So to reduce your risk of stings, do not confuse the insect into thinking you are a flower. That means:

- Dress in solid, neutral colors such as white or khaki.
- Stay away from floral patterns and floral colors like yellow, hot pink, orange, and green.
- Don't use scented products that may draw the insects near as does the scent of a flower. Avoid perfume and scented personal products such as soaps, sunscreen, hair care products, and body powders.
- Don't wear sandals in which a stinging insect could be trapped; wear closed-toe shoes such as sneakers instead.

If you're having a cookout or picnic, keep food covered until it's time to eat. Fresh fruit and soft drinks draw insects near. Uncovered garbage after the meal is particularly attractive to yellow jackets.

If stinging insects are nearby, stand still or move very slowly away from them. Don't swing your arms or move quickly because those motions can provoke an attack. Never crush an insect because that could release a special "alarm scent" that will mobilize nearby insects—particularly yellow jackets—to attack.

## SELF-CARE

If you are stung, remain calm. If you're with someone else who is stung, help maintain a calm atmosphere while you check out the situation. Slowly leave the area without swinging your arms. Resist the urge to try to swat the insects away.

Look at the site of the sting. If a stinger is visible, the sting came from a bee. These stingers can pump venom into the skin for a few minutes, so get rid of it. Try to flick the stinger with your fingernail, or scrape it away with something stiff such as a credit card or ID badge. Pull it out only if the other methods don't work.

There are two types of reactions to a sting: local, meaning limited to the skin, and systemic, meaning a response that affects the whole body. Systemic responses are the kind that should have you off to the ER.

Treat a local reaction with whatever is most handy. It is true that a meat tenderizer paste helps draw out the venom; add just enough water to the powder to make a paste (typically a few drops of water to a teaspoon of powder). Apply the paste to the area of the sting. Be sure to look for a tenderizer that contains papain, which is the enzyme that will help neutralize the venom.

To help relieve the redness, swelling, and itching of a sting:

- Wash the area with soap and water (after removing the stinger, if necessary).
- Apply cold compresses, or ice from a cooler if that's all that's nearby (try to wrap the ice in a cloth so you're not putting it directly on the skin, which could cause frostbite).
- Take a pain reliever of your choice, if needed.
- Use anti-inflammatory creams or local anesthetics for additional relief, as needed.

## LISTEN UP!

If you or a loved one has had a serious allergic reaction to an insect sting in the past, be sure to ask your HCP for an emergency kit. And, here's another tip: if you do need rescue medication, make sure you ask for a prescription that will allow you to buy more than one. If an allergic person plays golf, an extra kit should be in the golf bag; it won't do any good in the glove compartment in the parking lot. If it's an adolescent or young adult, an extra kit should go out to the athletic fields with a trainer, teacher, or coach during gym class or for outdoor games (like soccer, baseball, or softball).

Insect stings don't have to be a part of your summer. Using common sense and dressing smartly can keep these pesky intruders at bay.

## CUTS AND SCRAPES

### NURSE'S NOTE

We've come a long way since first aid for cuts was biting on a bullet and pouring whiskey over the wound to clean it! Both medical and nursing researchers have been studying the best way to care for wounds in hospitalized patients, and now you can follow that research-based approach when caring for yourself and your family at home.

### GET THEE TO THE ER

Go to the ER if you've gotten a cut and . . .

- Blood is spurting out.
- Bleeding does not stop after five minutes—by the clock—of firm direct pressure on the cut (without lifting the gauze every minute to see how it's doing, tempting as that may be).
- There's a good chance that the wound contains dirt, glass, or metal fragments, even though you can't see them.
- You've cut your hand or finger and are having trouble flexing or extending your fingers.
- The wound is a deep puncture wound, such as from stepping on a nail or other penetrating object.
- The cut is from a bite—human or animal.

## CALL YOUR HEALTH CARE PROVIDER

Before a noncritical injury occurs, known how your HCP prefers to handle it—in the office (so you can skip the ER or urgent care center altogether), at a walk-in center, or at the ER. Call first if:

- The cut looks closed and seems to have stopped bleeding, but then repeatedly opens back up when you try to resume your activities. This is particularly important if the cut is on your hand.
- The edges of the cut don't come together but you're not bleeding heavily.
- You have any conditions such as diabetes that can affect healing.

### Did You Know?

*Stitches* have been around a long time. Some HCP use only stitches. Others use them primarily in areas that need a very strong closure (such as on your hand). A very deep cut may need a layer of stitches under the skin surface to repair deeper tissues and another layer to close the skin.

*Staples* have become very popular to close surgical incisions. We also use them in the ER to close cuts when cosmetic result is not critical, such as on the scalp, where hair will cover any scar. Staples are quick and easy to put in. Both stitches and staples will have to be removed after a certain number of days, based on the location of the cut and how deep it is.

*Tissue glues* are gaining popularity as more research studies show that the cosmetic results (even on the face) are at least as good as, and in some cases better than, the results you'll get with stitches. Ask if it's an option where you go for closure of a cut. The glue is not removed; it wears off on its own.

*Butterflies* are the common name for adhesive bandages that can be used if the cut is not too deep, or the location is "out of the way" such as on the upper arm or back. Many people call these "butterfly" bandages because of their shape. These, too, will wear off on their own.

Also call if you have any signs of infection or concerns after stitches, staples, or glue have been used to close the cut.

## TECHNICALLY SPEAKING . . .

Injuries to the skin heal when new skin cells grow up from the bottom of the wound and fill in the cut. If a scab is present, oxygen can't get to that area of new skin growth as easily to help healthy

 **Frequently Asked Questions**

**Q.** *Are stitches really made from cat's guts?*
**A.** No, stitches are not made from catgut. Most used today are made from a special man-made, threadlike material. Original catgut was made from bovine intestines in the 1800s, and was favored because the stitches would dissolve after a period of time. It has been taken off the market in the United Kingdom, France, Germany, Spain, Austria, and Japan in favor of synthetic materials.

**Q.** *Is there a "time limit" for getting stitches?*
**A.** Yes, after about six to eight hours, the HCPs in the ER won't be able to use stitches or staples to close a cut. By that time, too many bacteria will have entered the wound and closing it increases the chance of infection. So if you cut yourself slicing vegetables for dinner, don't wait till morning to think about stitches. By then it will be too late.

**Q.** *How do I know if I need a tetanus shot?*
**A.** You need a tetanus shot if:

1. You can't remember when you last had one.
2. You have an injury and it has been more than five years since the last one.
3. It has been more than ten years since your last booster.

cells develop, which will slow healing. In addition, if the cells aren't growing in optimal conditions, they won't look like regular skin tissue—a condition called a scar.

## NURSE'S WISDOM

- Hydrogen peroxide should never be used to clean a cut. However, it can be used to get dried blood off uninjured skin adjacent to the cut. To get dried blood out of hair, dilute the hydrogen peroxide in warm water half and half, dampen the hair with the solution, and then comb through it.
- Some antibiotic ointments today have an anesthetic, or numbing medicine, mixed in to reduce pain. Check with the pharmacist at your pharmacy or discount store to help you select the right product for your particular needs. Look for pramoxine, a local anesthetic, in the list of ingredients.
- Don't be alarmed if cuts on the forehead or scalp bleed a lot since there are many superficial blood vessels in this area. Be calm, take a deep breath, and try to get a good look at the actual cut. You will probably be surprised at how small and manageable it is. If it's more than you think you can handle on your own, call your HCP or go to the ER.
- Don't hesitate to come to the ER because you're embarrassed about the way you injured yourself. Believe me, people who work in the ER have seen just about everything. We need a truthful explanation of your injury so that we can treat it properly and take any needed precautions against infection.
- Liquid Bandage® is a consumer version of Dermabond®, the tissue glue used by HCP. Liquid Bandage has less bond strength, so it's not meant to replace a trip to the HCP (and it won't stick your fingers together). It's great for small nicks and cuts, such as paper cuts, that you want to keep covered, and scrapes over areas that are almost impossible to bandage, such as elbows, knees, and knuckles.

## SELF-CARE

A survey by the Wound Care Resource Center of Johnson & Johnson (the makers of Band-Aid® brand bandages) found:

- Nearly half of the people surveyed don't routinely clean cuts.
- 70% don't treat their cuts and scrapes with an antibiotic ointment.
- 60% don't use a bandage to protect a cut or scrape.
- 72% think it's best to let a wound air out and form a scab.

The best way to care for cuts and scrapes is an easy-to-remember, three-step process:

**1. Clean.** The first thing to do for a cut or scrape is to clean it to prevent an infection. In the ER, we use equipment to squirt fluid on the cut or scrape and flush away dirt or germs. This is called irrigating and is the most effective cleansing technique. At home, you can wash the cut or scrape with soap under strong running water. Or look for plastic bottles of antiseptic that allow you to clean a cut or scrape by squirting the antiseptic out of the container.

Read the label of any antiseptic you choose. Benzalkonium chloride is an effective antiseptic that kills viruses and bacteria. Research shows that hydrogen peroxide damages cells when put directly on injured skin, so it's not a good choice.

Try not to dab or wipe the cut or scrape with moist gauze. Dabbing can push dirt into the skin. Wiping with a gauze pad or washcloth can damage delicate injured skin. Flush or irrigate the cut or scrape, and let it air dry before you go to the next step.

**2. Treat.** Research has taught us that preventing infection is very important to shorten healing time, lessen complications, and reduce scarring. After the cut or scrape is cleaned, apply antibiotic ointment. You have a number of product choices today. You can buy a tube of ointment and apply it to the injury (but don't touch the tip of the tube to the skin so the tip stays sterile). Or you can buy special Band-Aids® that have antibiotic ointment already on the pad.

3. **Protect.** If you think the best way for a cut or scrape to heal is to allow a scab to form, you're not alone. Most people think that's the best thing to do. But if a scab forms, it blocks the body's ability to make new skin cells. These new cells heal the cut or scrape and reduce the risk of a scar. Scabs actually *prolong* the healing process! Scabs also tend to get bumped, picked, or torn, which can lead to re-injury or more scarring.

Both medical and nursing research show that keeping a wound covered and moist and preventing scabs is the best way to heal the skin and reduce scarring. We have completely changed how we treat people with serious leg ulcers or bedsores as a result of this new information. You can do the same at home.

Keep the cut or scrape covered until you see that new skin has formed and healing is well on its way. Take the bandage off once a day for a bath or shower, and then reapply the antibiotic ointment and bandage for the rest of the day.

## LISTEN UP!

Keep the injury covered with a bandage for about seven to ten days, or until you can see the new skin forming to heal the injury. Check each day for signs of infection, including swelling, redness, red streaks going away from the injury toward the body, fluid or pus draining from the area, increasing pain, and sometimes fever.

If you've seen a HCP:

▪ Follow the instructions given to you. Ask for them in writing.
▪ If you have stitches or staples holding the wound edges together, have them removed when the HCP tells you to. Don't delay. Keeping them in longer won't help healing, increases the risk of scarring, and can make removing the staples or sutures much more difficult for us (and uncomfortable for you).

■ Keep the area dry except when showering. Don't take baths, swim, or soak in the hot tub while the stitches or staples are in place. After showering, pat the area dry and cover with a bandage (unless it is on your head, you don't need to try to put a Band-Aid® on your hair).

Three simple steps—clean, treat, and protect—will get you well on the way down the road to quicker healing with less scarring.

## SPRAINS AND STRAINS

### NURSE'S NOTE

At some point, just about everyone has a sprain or strain. A sprain occurs when the ligaments in the joints that hold bones together are overstretched (mild sprain) or torn (severe sprain). A sprain is an injury. The joints most commonly affected are the ankles, wrists, and knees.

A strain is a muscle that's been stretched too far. Muscle strains are a normal part of everyday life, and can occur, for example, when doing spring activities after a relatively inactive winter. Strains most often affect the back, neck, or leg.

As a nurse who's taken care of thousands of people with sprains and strains, I can tell you that when people say, "My ankle is broken; I heard the snap," there is rarely a break on the X ray. Hearing a snap is more likely indicative of a ligament tear.

### GET THEE TO THE ER

You can treat many sprain and strain injuries at home, but if the sprain or strain is severe or there is a chance that a bone is broken, you'll need to get medical help. Go to your local ER or urgent care center if any of these conditions is present in the injured area:

- A pain so severe that you are unable to bear weight.
- A pale, dusky blue color or lack of a pulse at the injured site or in the fingers or toes below the injury.
- An inability to move the limb.
- A feeling of numbness or unusually cold fingers or toes.
- An obvious deformity of the limb or massive swelling.

One note about numbness: I've taken care of a lot of injured people in the ER who felt numbness and tingling because they were hyperventilating from the pain and upset from the injury. If that's the only sign from this list, and the injured person is crying, breathing fast, or upset, numbness alone may not require a trip to the ER.

## CALL YOUR HEALTH CARE PROVIDER

- If symptoms are not beginning to improve after two to three days of appropriate self-care

## SELF-CARE

When the sprain or strain is in a joint such as the ankle or wrist, the treatment is the same: RICE—not Uncle Ben's, but Rest, Ice, Compression, and Elevation.

1. **Rest** means just that—not using the injured area. If you've injured your hand or wrist, rest means not using that hand to eat, write, type, carry things, or drive. For a knee, foot, or ankle injury, rest usually means using crutches for 24 to 72 hours, so that the injured area isn't bearing any of your body weight.

2. **Ice** means applying an ice or cold pack to reduce bruising and swelling. The standard routine is to put the ice on the injured site for 20 minutes and then take it off for 40 minutes. Ice should be your closest friend after a sprain or strain. It helps decrease the swelling that occurs in tissues after an injury. Less swelling means

less pain. In addition, ice will numb the area of injury, further reducing pain. You should start applying ice as soon as possible, but ice will still be helpful if you begin applying it up to 24 hours after the injury occurs.

**3. Compression** means using a stretchy bandage—for example, an ACE® wrap—that applies gentle, constant pressure to the injured area to limit swelling. Limit swelling, and you'll limit pain. A compression bandage will also provide protection for the skin when you apply ice, so you don't need to add a towel between the bandage and the ice.

Be sure to use the compression bandage properly. Always wrap from the injured area toward the heart. For the ankle, for example, start wrapping at the toes and wrap the bandage snugly (but not too tightly) around the ankle and a little ways up the leg. If you wrap the compression bandage toward the toes, on the other hand, blood and tissue fluid will collect in the toes, and swelling will worsen. The same goes for a wrist or hand injury. Start wrapping at the fingers and work the bandage up over the wrist and toward the elbow. Don't be afraid to loosen the bandage and rewrap if it feels too tight.

**4. Elevation** means keeping the injured area raised above the level of the heart to reduce swelling. Have you noticed a pattern? More swelling equals more pain.

Placing your sprained ankle on a footstool isn't true elevation. The proper technique would be lying flat on the couch with your foot up on about four pillows so the ankle is higher than your heart. (Be sure to have that TV remote control or juicy novel handy!)

If you follow these four steps for 24 to 48 hours, most mild to moderate strains and sprains should heal quickly. Typically, it takes a strain about a week to heal; a bad sprain can take three to four weeks. During this healing time, you'll need to limit your activities so you don't reinjure yourself.

If you have a broken bone, you'll probably wear a splint for a few days before a cast is applied to give the swelling time to decrease. RICE works with a splint, too.

Pain medication is best taken on a regular schedule (every so many hours as the label directs) for the first 24 to 48 hours after the injury so that you have a constant level of medicine in your blood. If you wait until you're in a lot of pain before taking anything, you'll be trying to catch up with the pain, and that's rarely successful.

Since strains and sprains cause significant inflammation, an anti-inflammatory drug such as ibuprofen, naproxen, or ketoprofen is a good first choice. Aspirin is also good if you can take it. Acetaminophen will not reduce inflammation as effectively. Do *not* increase the dose beyond the label's instructions if your pain is not relieved; instead, call your HCP to ask about a stronger prescription medicine. If you do get a prescription, ask if you can continue to take the OTC anti-inflammatory with the prescription pain pills.

Be aware that if ice packs are used improperly, frostbite can occur. Here are some important ice safety tips:

- Make sure there's something, such as a thin towel, (or the ACE® wrap) between the ice and your skin.
- Don't leave the ice pack on for more than 20 minutes.
- Don't go to sleep with the ice pack on.

## NURSE'S WISDOM

### Applying ice:
- Partially crushed ice cubes in a plastic bag will work.
- Check your freezer for a bag of frozen peas or corn. No kidding. These bags mold easily to the shape of your body and thus provide more constant and evenly distributed cold. You can also refreeze them for ongoing treatment of your injury. But if you use vegetables for first aid, they'll thaw so you shouldn't eat them afterward.
- Most drugstores carry chemical cold packs, which are portable and easy to use; you "activate" them and they become cold

within a minute or two. However, these are not reusable and a bit costly. They're best used for an on-the-go first aid kit.

■ You can make your own cold "slushy" packs. Mix one part water to one part rubbing alcohol. Place the solution in a plastic freezer bag and put it in your freezer. In a few hours, you'll have a partially frozen, shapeable ice pack.

■ Or use my favorite—those flaxseed-filled "snuggies" that you can put in the freezer. They are pliable, easy to use, and—an added bonus—often contain lavender or other nice-smelling ingredients for a little aromatherapy with your RICE.

### Applying compression bandages.

Before you apply a compression bandage, squeeze a finger- or toenail that will be beyond the wrap. After you squeeze it, the nail bed will turn white, and then should get pink as soon as you let go. This lets you know circulation is adequate. After you apply the wrap, squeeze the nail again. If it takes longer to turn pink, you've wrapped so tight, you're decreasing circulation. Loosen the bandage a bit. When it takes the same length of time for the nail to turn pink, you've got the wrap just right.

### Using crutches.

If you need crutches, make sure they are fitted properly—by someone who knows how to do this—to your height and the distance between your armpits and your feet. If the crutches are too tall, pressure can damage the huge bundle of nerves that runs through the armpits. You can also cause nerve damage if you lean on the crutches, allowing your body weight to rest on the top of the crutch under your arms. If the crutches are too short you'll always be bent over, which can easily injure your lower back.

With the proper size crutches, your weight should be on your hands on the hand grip of each crutch. A crutch grip is usually made of rubber, and after the first day, your hands will smell of rubber and the grip will just plain smell from the oils and sweat from your skin. To avoid this, try this tip that I used when I was on crutches for many months in the seventh grade:

- Fold a washcloth in half and wrap it around the hand grip.
- Tape it in place with regular adhesive tape.
- Dust the washcloth with baby powder or other powder of your choice to reduce moisture.
- Change the washcloth as often as you like.

This allows you to have a fresh hand grip whenever you want one. You can go to a discount store and buy an inexpensive large package of washcloths just for your crutches. The terry cloth also reduces the chance your sweaty hand will slip on the grip.

Finally, practice your technique in front of someone who knows what crutch-walking should look like so any errors can be corrected before you're on your own. Common problems include:

- Holding the crutches too far away from your sides; they should be almost touching your leg.
- Taking too big a "step" with the crutches out in front of your body; start by placing the crutches no more than six to eight inches in front of you, and then pivot your weight to your hands as you hop forward on your "good" leg.

# POISON CONTROL

## NURSE'S NOTE

Poison control is not just for people with kids. While 53% of poison exposures occur in children, more than 60% of poison fatalities occur in adults. Each year, U.S. poison control centers handle reports of more than two million poison exposures.

Repeat after me: **1-800-222-1222**. Throughout the United States, contacting the poison control center nearest you is that easy. You don't need to know the local number when you're on vacation or traveling on business. Dial this toll-free number, and you will automatically be connected to the nearest center. If you call on your cell phone, you may be connected to the center closest to your phone's home base. If you're someplace else, the poison expert can refer you to the center closest to where you are. Tape this number to your phone, and program it into speed dial.

## GET THEE TO THE ER

If the person is unconscious, having trouble breathing, or otherwise seriously injured, call emergency services first. While you wait for the ambulance to arrive, call 1-800-222-1222.

## INSIDER INFO

Calls to poison control are confidential, so don't ever hesitate to call. When you call, you'll speak to a poison expert. It's usually a nurse, but you could also talk with a physician, pharmacist, or toxicologist. They'll ask for your name and phone number so that they can call you back or send emergency services if you get disconnected.

Data collected by poison control centers are not tracked back to individuals; rather, they are used together to identify hazards, direct research, and help train the experts who staff poison control center hotlines nationwide. We all benefit from what's in the annual report compiled from this data. This information has led to product recalls, changes in product labeling, and more effective warnings on labels.

Poison control centers are a terrific resource. We call them from the ER whenever we need advice because the staff are the poison experts who can confirm if an exposure is or is not a poisoning. For example, they can tell you:

- If you've overdosed when you realize that the three multi-symptom cold remedies you've taken in the past four hours all contained acetaminophen (Tylenol).

- What to do if, while working on your car, some fluid splashes into your eye.
- What to do if concentrated pool chemicals went through a hole in your glove and got on your skin.
- What to do if you've inhaled a potentially poisonous gas (perhaps in the workplace or in your home workshop).
- What to do if you've been bitten or stung by a potentially poisonous creature.

## Frequently Asked Questions

Q. What will the poison control center ask when I call?

A. The person on duty will ask for the following information:

- Your name and the phone number from which you are calling (and sometimes the zip code of your current location for data analysis purposes).
- The affected person's age and approximate weight.
- Any signs or symptoms.
- The time the exposure occurred—for example, how many minutes or hours ago.
- The name of the substance (reading off the label is best if you have the original container).
- The amount of the substance that was swallowed, inhaled, or spilled (or a reasonable estimate).
- The affected person's health history, including any medicines taken regularly.

Q. What if the substance isn't really poisonous and it was all a mistake?

A. Better safe than sorry. If there's any doubt about a substance, call. If everything is okay, everyone will breathe a sigh of relief. There's no penalty for being cautious.

## TECHNICALLY SPEAKING . . .

Poisons' effects on the body are determined by what the poison is, how the person is exposed (if the poison is swallowed, breathed in, or splashed on the skin), and the amount or dose of poison (medications, for example, can be therapeutic in recommended doses but become a poison if taken in overdose). Poisons can:

- Irritate or burn the skin.
- Inflame or irritate delicate tissues from the mouth to the lungs if you inhale fumes or toxic gases.
- Damage lung tissue and cause severe breathing difficulty.
- Cause allergic reactions such as a skin rash, runny nose, and asthma symptoms.
- Cause drowsiness, headache, confusion, and disorientation that may lead to loss of consciousness.
- Make your muscles weak, which can even progress to paralysis.
- Make you sick to your stomach, with or without vomiting.
- Cause abnormal heart rhythms that can range from mild to life-threatening.
- Increase the risk of some cancers if there is long-term exposure to low levels of certain poisons.

## NURSE'S WISDOM

The best poison treatment is prevention:

- Always keep medicines and household chemicals in their original containers.
- Never, ever put anything that is not a beverage in a soda bottle.
- Use devices designed to limit a child's access to drawers and cabinets, but don't think these are like padlocks—chemicals and medicines should be stored in a high place not accessible to children.
- Never take medicine in the dark.

- Never combine cleaning agents; combining chlorine bleach and ammonia can create a toxic cloud.
- Put the national poison number on every phone in your house and program it into speed dial of your home, office, and cell phones.

## SELF-CARE

If the poisoning is serious, call the poison control center at 1-800-222-1222. The poison expert you reach will stay on the line with you while emergency medical services (EMS) are alerted. The expert will continue to talk with you until the EMS professionals arrive and will then speak to them on your telephone to provide any instructions needed for care during the ride to the hospital. Once you're on your way, the poison expert will call the ER to alert them that you are coming, and what they need to do when you arrive.

If the poisoning does not seem serious, call the poison control center anyway at 1-800-222-1222 so the poison expert can confirm your hunch. Depending on the exposure, self-care described below will happen before you call poison control if your self-care will limit exposure to the poison (such as flushing the skin) or after you call the center.

### Swallowed poison:
- Don't eat or drink until you've talked to a poison expert.
- Don't try to vomit unless the poison experts recommend that you do to empty your stomach. This is done less often nowadays.

### Inhaled poison:
- Get into fresh air right away—this could mean going indoors or outdoors, depending on the source of the poison.
- Avoid continuing to expose yourself or other people to the poison.

### Skin or eyes to poison:
- Take off any clothing that has poison on it.
- Continually flush the skin with plain water (from a hose,

shower, or faucet)—whatever is closest—until you've talked with a poison expert.

■ If the poison has gotten in an eye, flush the eye for about 20 minutes. Use a large cup, repeatedly fill it with lukewarm water, and pour it across the eye from the nose toward the ear. If you can, hold the eyelid open. You need to get the poison off the eye itself; pouring water across a closed eyelid won't do much good, but don't give up!

## LISTEN UP!

The good news is that 77% of exposures are treated with telephone advice only. Keys are:

■ Call whenever you suspect a poisoning; there's no penalty for a false alarm.
■ Have the container that held the poison with you at the phone if it is available and if doing so will not further expose you to poison.

Other than the first aid measures listed above, do *not* do anything on your own without consulting poison control. When it comes to poisonings, an ounce of prevention is worth far more than a pound of cure.

# HOME SAFETY

## NURSE'S NOTE

According to the National Safety Council, each year seven million Americans are disabled by injuries that occur in the home and 28,000 more die from home injuries. As an ER nurse, I can vouch for the fact that some of the more serious injuries I've treated have not been from car crashes, but from injuries that happened at home. The leading cause of home injury is fires and number two is falls.

Most people think about childproofing a home, but safety isn't only for kids—or seniors. Safety should be for everyone—whether you own your home, rent, or live in a temporary place such as a dormitory. The principles are the same everywhere. You may have less control over some items if you don't own the home, but that doesn't mean you can't raise a ruckus to improve the safety where you live to reduce injuries and save lives.

## COMMON HOME SAFETY ISSUES

### Electrical.

Older homes do not have ground fault circuit interrupters (GFCI). This device monitors electricity flowing through a circuit—typically an outlet near a water source in the bathroom, kitchen, laundry area, or swimming pool. If there is an imbalance in the circuit, as may occur if an appliance plugged into a GFCI comes in contact with water, the GFCI will shut off the power, significantly reducing the risk of electrical injury.

Do not run electrical cords or extension cords across a walking area where someone could trip. Also resist the urge to try to hide a cord under a throw rug; if there's any heat buildup, a fire could start.

### Fall prevention.

Falls can cause serious injuries and death, and there are a number of places in a home where the risk is high. To prevent falls, take the following precautions:

- Use a nonslip mat on the bottom of the shower or tub unless it is one of the newer models that has a molded nonskid surface.
- Don't forget that a wet tile floor adjacent to the shower or tub can be just as dangerous if it's not covered. Use high-quality mats with rubber backings that will eliminate sliding.

- Never grab a towel rack for help getting out of the tub; it won't support your weight, and you'll fall.
- Add a handrail to steps in and out of the home. Even the three steps at the back door can lead to a nasty injury if you slip, there is no handrail to grab on to, and you land on cement.
- Resist the urge to pile the clean laundry high in the basket if you have to carry it upstairs to put it away. If you can't see, you're much more likely to fall.
- Place rubber backing underneath any throw rug to prevent it from slipping when you step on it. Likewise, clean up any liquid spills on wood, tile, or vinyl floors as soon as possible. Don't wax floors if it will make them slippery.
- And, as attractive as a glass coffee table may be in your decorating scheme, it's not a particularly safe choice. I have spent more hours that I can count with patients who've had hundreds of stitches because they slipped, tried to catch themselves by reflexively putting their hand out on the table, and instead broke the table's glass and sliced up their hand and arm.

**Fire safety.**
Smoke alarms are essential. People who die in house fires don't typically die from burns, but from inhaling smoke and toxic gases, often while they are sleeping. To ensure that your smoke alarms are effective, do the following:

- Choose battery-powered smoke detectors that will work whether or not you have electrical power in the building.
- *Replace*—don't just check—the batteries twice a year. Remember the phrase, "Change your clock, change your batteries." If you replace the batteries when you turn the clocks forward and backward, you should be protected. (And if you live in an area where the clocks don't change, you'll know when the rest of the country does it.)
- Test the batteries once a month to be sure they work.
- Place smoke detectors on each level of the home, and outside

each bedroom door if your home is that large, or if bedrooms are on different levels. Don't forget the basement if you have one.

Also follow these other fire safety tips:

- If you have a fireplace and chimney, have it professionally checked annually and cleaned if necessary to reduce the risk of a chimney fire.
- Keep portable heaters away from fabric such as billowing draperies.
- Never walk away when you're cooking on the stove, particularly if you are frying. If a fire occurs, smother it by putting a lid on the frying pan. If you don't have a cover, keep baking soda in the cabinet closest to the stove as a safety measure to smother a grease fire.
- Home fire extinguishers are inexpensive, lightweight, and easy to use. An area of high risk where you might place it is the kitchen; make sure it is positioned so that the person grabbing the fire extinguisher is moving toward an exit, not deeper into the room, in case the fire gets quickly out of control. If you have a wood stove or other areas in the home in which there is fire risk, you will need additional units.
- Don't forget the three words that were drilled into me (and probably you too) in grammar school: stop, drop, and roll. If your clothing or hair catches fire, stop—don't run—drop to the floor or ground, and roll around to smother the flame.
- Examine your home for evacuation routes. How would you and your family members get out in an emergency if the doors and staircase are blocked by flames? Be sure everyone knows the options, and establish a central location for everyone to meet outside in case you are separated while you get out.

Carbon monoxide (CO) poisoning is another safety threat, especially in cold climates at the beginning of the heating season. People can seal off the furnace during summer projects and not realize it.

When heating fuel prices rise, people want a "tighter house," and that can trap carbon monoxide as well as heat. To prevent CO poisoning, experts recommend that you install at least one CO detector near bedrooms. I'd suggest another closer to the furnace or wood stove if you have one so that you will get an earlier warning than waiting for the gas to reach the bedroom area.

### Home improvement.

The home improvement industry has grown from sales of $92.6 billion in 1991 to a projected $254.8 billion in 2007. More work on homes, however, means more injuries. Here's what you need to do to stay safe:

- Practice safe laddering. That means don't climb on a ladder—indoors or outdoors—when you're all alone if no one could tell if you've fallen. If you're working on the front gutters and your house is on a busy street, that's one thing, but if you are hanging wallpaper in the staircase on a weekend and live alone, who would know if you fell? People pooh-pooh me all the time, but I have taken care of too many people—of all ages—who've fallen and lain on the floor for two days until someone noticed they didn't answer the phone or didn't pick up the mail. Also, position the ladder properly, with firm support and at an appropriate angle. Slip a cordless phone in your pocket or tool belt so you can call for help if a mishap occurs.
- Use protective clothing, goggles, heavy gloves, and ear coverings when appropriate. I want to scream when I see men working with chainsaws in their yards in the summertime wearing only sandals and a pair of shorts! Safety gear is not expensive; an eye injury can be. Also, don't wear loose clothing that could get caught in a power tool.
- Know what you're doing; read the instructions. Over 110,000 ER visits result from home improvement gone wrong, and 65% of those injuries involve a blade of some sort. If it's a blade versus skin, the blade always wins.

**Lighting.**

Night lights are not just for kids. We bought small units at the hardware store with two lights that plug into an electrical outlet. When there is power, the green light glows as a night light. If the power goes out, the bright white light, automatically comes on, and runs on batteries, as emergency lighting. Pull the unit out of the outlet, and it's a handy flashlight. The number you'll need will be based on your floor plan, but the convenience and safety can't be beat.

**Stairways.**

Make sure steps and staircases are well lit so you know how many steps there are and so you won't miss that all-important last step. This means the few steps to the front door as well as the staircase going upstairs or downstairs to the basement. Follow these important stairway safety tips:

- Place light switches at the top and bottom of staircases.
- Resist the urge to use the stairs as a storage space, thinking, "I'll just put this here to remember to take it upstairs." Magazines on stairs are particularly dangerous. I've done that, slipped and fell, and have the scars to prove it.
- Have handrails on both sides of all stairways for maximum safety.
- If the steps are smooth, add traction treads for gripping. Be careful with your footwear; socks on wood stairs are a recipe for disaster.
- If the basement steps and the floor are both cement, paint the bottom step so your depth perception will be enhanced and allow you to see where the step ends and the floor begins.

## LISTEN UP!

Most injuries in the home are preventable. A few simple steps that cost less than $100 will show you a huge return on investment in safety and injuries prevented. For example, a knife sharpener costs about $20 to

---

**❓ Frequently Asked Questions**

Q. *What if my landlord won't make safety improvements?*
A. Check with your town hall to see what safety measures are required for residential rental units. If your landlord does not meet your city or town regulations, make a report. An inspector might make a stronger impression than you and get those changes made. If it's a critical issue such as a smoke detector, put your own on the ceiling while you fight it out. Don't risk your life.

---

$30. Many people don't realize dull knives cause more injuries than sharp ones. Since you use more pressure to try to cut with a dull knife that doesn't glide through foods, you're more likely to slip. And the knife too dull to pierce the tomato skin can do a number on your hand.

# TRAVEL HEALTH AND SAFETY

## NURSE'S NOTE

When you are traveling, plan ahead, stay alert, use common sense, and trust your gut so you won't be a target for crime. Know what your health insurance will and won't cover when you're away from home; believe it or not, many policies are much more liberal about covering ER visits when you're 1,000 miles from home since they can't require that you see your PCP first.

## GET THEE TO THE ER

If you are in a strange town and you get sick, particularly if you are traveling by yourself, go to the ER sooner than you would consider going at home. At least then you will have an ER nurse looking after you rather than risking being stranded in a hotel room.

## CALL YOUR HEALTH CARE PROVIDER

- If you're traveling outside the United States to get the latest information about recommended immunizations for the area to which you're traveling and any other health bulletins.
- Particularly if you have any chronic health conditions to find a health care provider where you're traveling.
- If you're going someplace sunny and warm to learn if any of your medications will make you sensitive to the sun.
- If you're traveling to a place that is particularly hot or humid or cold to ask about the best way to store prescription meds or your first aid kit.

## COMMON TRAVEL SAFETY ISSUES

### Air travel.
When you're flying, dress for safety. Stay away from clothes made from nylon and polyester fibers, such as pantyhose, because they burn easily. Nix the heels in case you need to move in a hurry. Stick with cotton, wool, denim, or leather clothing. Long sleeves and long pants, cotton socks, and flat shoes are ideal.

### Cruise ship travel.
The Centers for Disease Control has a Vessel Sanitation Program through which it inspects passenger ships that stop at any U.S. ports to reduce the risk of the spread of communicable diseases. The report, commonly called "The Green Sheet," is available at the Web site listed under Web Resources, or you can get a copy by fax by calling 1-888-232-6789 and requesting document 510051. You can search the online database for detailed information about particular ships.

## Frequently Asked Questions

**Q.** *How much medicine should I take with me?*
**A.** Being one who hates to check a bag, I never want to take something I don't absolutely need when I travel, but in recent years, I have learned to plan for delays. If you require daily medication, take twice as much as you'd need if you experienced no delays on your trip.

**Q.** *Is there anything else I need to take?*
**A.** Depending on how far you're going and how long you'll be gone, consider the following:

* A paper that lists your blood type, a contact person not traveling with you in case of emergency, immunizations and dates, allergies, and brief medical history including current health conditions and medications (particularly with generic names).
* Health insurance information, including the name and address of the company.
* Trip insurance information.
* A copy of your eyeglass prescription (and ideally, an extra pair of glasses).

## Hotel stays.

If you tend to be allergic, bring a few of your own pillowcases with you if you don't have room for your own pillow. An OTC antihistamine will not only keep allergic symptoms at bay, but can also help you sleep in an unfamiliar place.

## NURSE'S WISDOM

### Air travel:

■ People on long trips have been known to develop blood clots in their legs. These clots can break off and go to the lung, which can be serious—even deadly. You're at risk for what is dubbed "economy class syndrome" if you don't drink much water, if you have drinks containing alcohol, and if you don't regularly get up during the flight to stretch your legs. Ask your HCP about taking aspirin before your trip to help reduce blood clotting, skip the alcohol, drink plenty of water, and get up often. And don't cross your legs when you're in your seat.

■ Every in-flight magazine I've seen in the last year has added health tips, including exercises you can do while seated to enhance circulation. Look for these tips when you fly.

### Airport security and your health:

■ If you have a condition that prevents your shoes from being removed—because they are attached to braces or a prosthesis, for example—you cannot be forced to remove them; alternative security measures can be used such as moving a wand over your feet.

■ If you need to sit before, or at some point during, the screening process (such as if you have to go through additional screening after passing through the metal detector), the rules say you can sit. Speak up and let one of the screeners know, and be sure to keep an eye on your valuables.

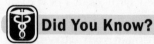 **Did You Know?**

Researchers tested 348 patients with pacemakers or implanted defibrillators to see if airport metal detectors interfered with proper functioning of these lifesaving heart devices. No interference was detected; the metal in the device will set off the metal detector, however. Therefore, Medtronic, the company that makes many of these devices, advises people who have them to ask that the handheld wand used for follow-up screening be kept away from the front of the chest as a safety precaution.

■ If you have a medical condition that requires syringes or other
sharp medical equipment, it can be kept in your carry-on baggage provided you notify the screener you have equipment
with you that will need to be checked and that your medication is labeled from the pharmacy (save the vial or box where
the label is located and bring it with you). As an extra measure of validation, it can't hurt to have a letter signed by your
HCP on letterhead that states:

John Palmer is under my care for a medical condition that requires
him to take medicine by injection. He needs to carry syringes and
needles, lancets to obtain a blood sample for testing, test supplies,
and a container for used equipment.

OR

Melissa O'Brien receives medication through an implanted pump located under the skin of her abdomen. She must carry syringes, additional medication, and back-up intravenous equipment.

If you want the letter to go into detail about the nature of your
medical condition, that's up to you. Key point: don't surprise
the screeners; it can look like you are trying to sneak something through. If you must carry used syringes, it's best to put
them in your checked baggage.

■ If a security screener needs to go through your carry-on bag,
warn him or her that medical equipment is in your bag and ask
if you may remove it to prevent them from getting injured. You
are not supposed to reach in your bag after they have started
the inspection process, so make the offer as a way to protect
the screener. Don't just reach in your bag.

■ If you pack any medical equipment, use see-through plastic or
mesh bags so screening goes faster.

■ If you have a pacemaker, artificial joint, or other prosthesis, particularly if there's metal that will set off the detector, carry your

medical ID card. Check with your HCP or the manufacturer to make sure it is safe for you to go through a metal detector and if a screening wand can cause the device to malfunction.

■ If you need a pat-down, particularly if the pat-down is related to a medical condition, recent surgery, implant, or prosthesis, you have the right to ask for personal screening in a private area. Your medical condition should remain confidential between you and Transportation Security Administration (TSA) personnel during the screening process.

■ If you need assistance to get to the gate, or need to accompany a friend or family member, you'll need an authorized companion gate pass from the ticket counter that will allow an additional person through security with the ticketed passenger. It's not a big deal and will ease everyone's mind if you can stay together through to the gate, particularly in a huge airport.

■ If you have any problems, contact the TSA directly at their hotline at 1-866-289-9673.

## Back pain and travel:

■ If you don't have back pain before your trip, it's easy to end up with pain along the way if you don't follow some precautions:

1. Get luggage with wheels. (How did we survive before this invention?)

2. Get someone to help you put a carry-on bag in the overhead compartment on a plane if you cannot place it under the seat in front of you, the more back-friendly location.

3. Support your lower back while seated in a car, plane, or train with a rolled up blanket, towel, or pillow.

4. Get up and stretch; walk regularly.

5. Carry plastic bags with you; if your back acts up while you're

traveling, you can fill one with ice and put it between your back and the seat.

**6.** Change position slowly, and don't twist while carrying luggage.

**7.** A tip for a skycap or bellman is a small price to pay to reduce the risk of back pain while you travel.

## SELF-CARE

■ When traveling, carry a basic first aid kit with you, keeping in mind that if you're flying, tweezers and scissors aren't allowed in the cabin, but are fine in checked bags. You can make your own kit with a heavy-duty plastic freezer bag and small samples of bandages, gauze, and tape; antibiotic ointment; a pain reliever/fever medicine; remedies for diarrhea, constipation, and motion sickness; a decongestant (good for "airplane ears," described on p. 15); an antihistamine; and an alcohol-based mouthwash that can double as an antiseptic if necessary. Add a 2 or 4 ounce bottle of hand sanitizer and you're all set.

■ Also when traveling, bring your medication, in a carry-on bag that is with you at all times. It's best to keep medicines in the original prescription bottles; if you're traveling overseas, it's essential. Don't forget to bring any regular OTC medicines as well. Carry your medicine list (see p. 210). If you are overseas, the generic names will remain the same, but the brand names will differ. Double check about any foods or beverages you should avoid where you're traveling. If you forget a medicine, you can usually have a prescription transferred for a small number of pills to get you through your trip; just call your home pharmacy.

■ Don't forget the regular things you'd do at home, such as use sunscreen, drink plenty of water, and put the national poison control number—1-800-222-1222—on speed dial on your cell phone.

- Know that travel often slows your intestines down and that constipation is common when you're away from home, so be prepared. (See constipation remedies on p. 145.)
- At your destination, know if you can dial 911 for emergencies or if there is another number, and what that number is.

## LISTEN UP!

Don't carry all of your money, identification, or medicines in one place such as your pocketbook or wallet. Particularly if you're traveling with someone else, spread the items around so if something gets lost or you're the target of a pickpocket, you won't lose everything.

Photocopy everything of importance—credit cards, passport, insurance card, driver's license, and so on—before you leave and keep one copy with you in a different place than the original items. Also give a copy to a trusted friend or relative not traveling with you, who could fax you the info or read it to you over the phone if you need it.

Not every community in the United States uses the 911 system for emergencies. If you are staying at a friend's or relative's house, or renting a vacation house, ask if they use 911 where they live. If not, put the local emergency number by every phone.

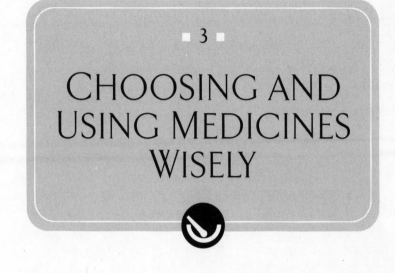

■ 3 ■

# CHOOSING AND USING MEDICINES WISELY

# WHAT YOU MUST KNOW ABOUT EVERY PRESCRIPTION

## NURSE'S NOTE

As the health-care system changes, we, as consumers, need to change along with it. I remember when there were one or two family doctors in town and one pharmacy owned by the pharmacist. The pharmacist knew the doctors and the patients, and it wasn't so important that patients kept tabs on everything because a system of checks and balances was already in place.

Today, the built-in safeguards are not as automatic as they once were, so now you need to step up and take personal responsibility for your own safety when it comes to prescription and OTC medicines. Here's how:

- Be sure you know why you are taking any prescription medication. Before your HCP writes the prescription, ask why you need to take the medicine and how it will help you so you can monitor the effects.
- Whenever you can, have all of your prescriptions filled at the

same pharmacy so there is a record of all of your medicines and the pharmacy computer can automatically check for any interactions. If you must use a mail-away service, give your neighborhood pharmacist a list of all of your drugs to keep in the computer for interaction checking when you need a short-term medicine, such as an antibiotic.

■ If you take more than one medicine for the same condition, be sure you know which drug to take when. For example, there are asthma inhalers that should be used every day, regardless of symptoms, and there are other inhalers that should only be used for shortness of breath.

■ If you have taken corticosteroid drugs such as prednisone, cortisone, or Medrol for more than two weeks in the past two years, be sure and tell all your health providers including dentists and anesthesia providers. Be sure and keep the name, dose, and length of time you took the pills on your medicine list (see p. 210).

■ If you have people in your house to clean, house sit, or walk your dogs when you aren't there, remember that some prescription medicines have street and recreational value—particularly pain medicine, sedatives, and tranquilizers. You may want to store these drugs in a special, out-of-the-way location. I include this tip because the Tylox prescribed for me when I had a surgery was missing when I needed it after a follow-up procedure. Looking back, we put things together, figured out how it vanished, and changed the locks.

## CALL YOUR HEALTH CARE PROVIDER

■ If you experience side effects that are so troublesome you want to stop taking the medicine.
■ If you don't think the medicine is working.
■ If you don't think you need to take the medicine any longer.
■ If you have concerns about cost, and want to find out if there is a less expensive drug that will do the job for you.

■ If you are tempted to stop taking medicine. Don't just skip the medicine without checking in to share your concerns and explore alternatives.

## INSIDER INFO

Let's break the code right here and now. Here's how a prescription is written:

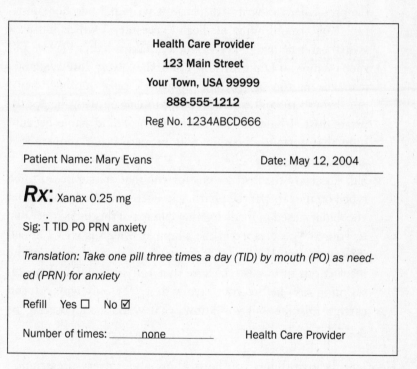

**Health Care Provider**
**123 Main Street**
**Your Town, USA 99999**
**888-555-1212**
Reg No. 1234ABCD666

Patient Name: Mary Evans          Date: May 12, 2004

**Rx:** Xanax 0.25 mg

Sig: T̄ TID PO PRN anxiety

*Translation: Take one pill three times a day (TID) by mouth (PO) as needed (PRN) for anxiety*

Refill    Yes ☐    No ☑

Number of times: _____none_____          Health Care Provider

Here's what each item means:

■ **Patient name:** Your name is written here. As an added safety measure, if you are mailing your prescription away to be filled or are going to a large pharmacy, add your date of birth so you can be sure they know which Mary Evans you are. Adding your address can't hurt, either.

■ **Rx:** This is the name of the medication and the strength. The form is a pill or tablet unless otherwise noted as, for example, a suppository, liquid, or ointment. The medication can be written as the brand name or the generic (or chemical) name. Today, most insurance plans call for the pharmacist to fill the prescription with the generic form of the drug if one is available, because it is less expensive. All states allow this. If there is a particular reason you need the brand name formulation, the prescriber can write "dispense as written," "do not substitute," or "brand name medically necessary," which means a switch can't be made. For example, I take a half a Flexeril pill each evening. If I take a whole pill of the lowest dose available, it makes me too sleepy. But, the generic pills crumble when I put them in the pill cutter. In order to end up with the appropriate dose, I have to pay extra for the brand name because only that form can cut in half properly. (For more about generic drugs, see p. 204.)

■ **Sig:** These are the instructions for you that are supposed to be typed on the label at the pharmacy. There is a whole shorthand vocabulary used in medicine that can make this indecipherable to you, as you can see in the example, which is why I added the translation. If your HCP doesn't have time to write out the instructions in English, be sure that you know what that prescription says before you leave with it. The only way you can catch a mistake is if you know what you are supposed to be getting.

Here are the five things you must know about every prescription you receive:

1. Name of the medicine (brand name and generic name) and strength (usually in milligrams).

2. How many pills to take (or whatever the dosing form is).

3. How often you should take the medicine. Does three times a day mean breakfast, lunch, and dinner, or is it important to try to separate doses eight hours apart?

4. Do you take the medicine only when you have a certain symptom, such as for anxiety, as in our example, or do you need to take it daily, on a regular schedule? The letters "PRN" (from the Latin *pro re nata*) stand for "when needed" or "when necessary" and should be followed by specific instructions such as "PRN for pain" or "PRN for itching" or "PRN for diarrhea." If the label just says, "Take one pill three times a day as needed," You may forget precisely why the drug was prescribed.

5. Check on the refill status so you know whether the prescription can be refilled or if your HCP wants to talk with you or see you before ordering a refill. Some drugs that have the potential for abuse have limits on refills without a brand new written prescription, and prescriptions for some drugs expire—whether you have the written prescription on your refrigerator with a magnet or if you call in for a refill. The pharmacist will tell you if you need to get a new prescription. You need to keep track to allow extra time for a new prescription so you don't run out of pills.

## TECHNICALLY SPEAKING . . .

Almost every insurance plan has what is called a "formulary." This is a list of drugs it prefers that you use. Most of the time, it is because the formulary contains the drugs that cost the insurance company less. Sometimes, however, it is because a particular drug is more likely to be taken as directed when compared with another drug. For example, the antibiotic Zithromax is more expensive as a brand-name drug than other generic options, but the great thing about Zithromax is that you take two pills to start and then one pill a day for only four more days. You're much more likely to follow

## ? Frequently Asked Questions

**Q.** *Are generic drugs really as good as brand-name drugs? I don't think generic cola tastes as good as Coke.*

**A.** Brand-name drugs usually belong to only one pharmaceutical company that spent all the money on the research to invent the drug and test it for years before earning approval from the FDA to release it for general use by patients. The company has a patent that gives them exclusive rights to sell that drug for, on average, 9 to 12 years. Once that patent expires, other drug manufacturers are then permitted to make the drug. When a drug is produced and sold under the chemical name, it is called a generic drug. A generic is a chemical clone of the branded drug. Since the companies that are making these plain drugs did not invest the time and money in the research required to invent a new drug, they charge less for each pill. Savings amount to about 52% of total drug cost when a person switches from brand-name to generic medications.

The FDA has a separate Office of Generic Drugs that oversees manufacturing to make sure generics meet established standards, which include:

- Same active ingredients shown to work the same way in the body as the brand-name drug (does not get in the bloodstream any faster or slower than the brand, for example).
- Same quality control measures, purity, strength, and chemical stability.
- Same pharmaceutical manufacturing standards.

Generic pills will usually be different in shape and color than their brand-name counterparts. In rare cases, some people may require the brand name instead of generic because they are allergic to the generic pill's *inactive* ingredients such as coloring or coating. About half of the generic drugs on the market today are made in the very same facilities as their brand-name cousins.

Q. *My doctor prescribed Prevacid for my heartburn, but when I got to the pharmacy, I was given a bottle of pills called Prilosec. Is this what's meant by "generic substitution"?*

A. No! Generic substitution is when a chemical clone is provided instead of the brand-name drug. However, it is the same drug. Prevacid and Prilosec are similar in effect but completely different drugs. Technically, this practice is called "therapeutic substitution" because it is changing to a drug that has a similar effect, but it's not substituting a plain label generic for the chemically identical brand-name drug. Many insurance companies routinely require pharmacies to ask for permission to change drugs considered to be equivalent in their action on the body because they want you to get the less expensive drug to keep costs down. If you're not happy about the change, contact your HCP; permission had to come from your prescriber's office in order for the switch to happen. And don't blame pharmacists; they're stuck in the middle.

those instructions and take all four pills instead of having to remember to take a different antibiotic pill three or four times a day for ten days. In this case, it costs less in the long run to treat an infection properly the first time even if the pills cost a bit more.

If your employer offers choices among insurance plans and you and your family members take prescription medicine every day, be sure to ask for the formularies of the different plans before you make your choice. You should be able to get a printed list or the Web site where the drugs are listed. Some plans won't cover drugs that aren't on the formulary list at all (meaning you have to pay the entire cost out of your pocket); other plans will require a higher co-payment to get the "nonpreferred" drug.

Your out-of-pocket costs may be significantly different under various plans if you and members of your family take medicines on a daily basis for conditions such as asthma, high blood pressure, migraine headaches, or allergies. If you have a choice of plans, sit down and do the math before you make your choice of health plans. One plan may cost less per pay period, but you may see it will cost

## Did You Know?

Nursing research has examined why some people are able to follow treatment plans and others have more trouble. Our knee-jerk reaction is to teach people more about their medication and condition, but we may be missing the boat. One study of men with high blood pressure identified key factors that play a role in whether a patient will follow a prescribed treatment plan. Think about whether any of these are barriers for you:

- How do you define health and illness? Do you need to feel sick before you'll take medicine?
- Does taking medicine affect your self-image and make you feel less strong?
- Are you reluctant to seek health care or have a prescription filled because you worry about protection of your privacy?
- What support systems do you have?
- Do you feel like your health problems are your fault and don't deserve treatment?
- Does your HCP take your life circumstances into account when developing a treatment plan?

If any of these ring true for you, take the lead and share your thoughts with your HCP. Together, you can explore your treatment options and come up with a plan that feels right for your beliefs and lifestyle.

more out of your pocket for medicines than another plan with a higher initial cost. Look at the overall costs—not just how much comes out of the paycheck.

## NURSE'S WISDOM

### Preventing medication errors:

■ Before you leave your HCP's office with a prescription, review it so you know what the drug is, why it is prescribed, how to take it, how you'll know if it's working, and any special considerations relating to the medicine.

■ Ask your HCP to write why the medicine is prescribed on the prescription itself. Take these examples: Celexa is an antidepressant and Celebrex is for arthritis; Zantac is for heartburn and Zyrtec is for allergies. If your HCP has poor handwriting, but wrote "Zyrtec for allergy symptoms" or "Celebrex for joint pain," it virtually eliminates the possibility that the pharmacist could confuse similar drug names because the handwriting is so hard to read. It will also help you keep your medicines straight if the label is typed that way.

■ Write a list of your medicines and carry a copy with you in your wallet or purse. (See p. 210 for a sample format you can photocopy and fill out or download a copy from www.nursenotebook.com.) Whenever you visit a HCP, ask someone in the office to make a copy of your list. Then give it to your HCP, review it with him or her, and ask that it be put in the medical record. That way, you can keep your record up to date, particularly if you are getting medicines from more than one HCP. Why should you list both generic and brand names? In case your medicine becomes available in generic form, you'll recognize the name. Be sure to include OTC medicines too. Here is an example:

| BRAND NAME | GENERIC NAME | DOSE (mg) | TIMES PER DAY | WHEN | FOR WHAT CONDITION | PRESCRIBER |
|---|---|---|---|---|---|---|
| None | atenolol | 25 mg | 1 | Bedtime | High Blood Pressure | Duff |
| Lipitor | atorvastatin | 10 mg | 1 | Bedtime | High cholesterol | Duff |
| Zyrtec | cetirizine | 10 mg | 1 | Symptoms | Allergies | McHugh |
| None | aspirin | 81 mg | 1 | Bedtime | Prevent heart attack | Duff |

■ Check every new prescription you get. First, make sure it's your name on the bottle and that you didn't get someone else's by mistake. If it's a refill, check the new pills against the old ones to see if they match. If they don't, have both pill bottles handy so you can provide any information from the labels, and call the pharmacy. Tell the pharmacist (and be sure to ask to speak with the pharmacist) that your pills look different and you're concerned there might be a mistake. It could be as simple as a change to a different generic manufacturer, or you may have caught an error. Every time this has happened to me, it was a change to a different generic manufacturer, but a phone call is a very simple safety check for you to make.

## Saving money on prescription:

- If you or someone you know has trouble paying for medicine, tell your HCP. Most prescribers don't take price into account when they write a prescription unless you bring it up. Don't be embarrassed; it is far more important to have food, shelter, *and* your medicine rather than having to choose which necessity you'll spend your money on.
- If your HCP is prescribing a new medicine, ask for a week's worth of samples to start. There's no need to buy a 90-day supply until you know you don't have side effects that would require a change of medicines. Otherwise, buying in quantity is usually a better way to save money.
- Pharmacies' expiration date on the prescription label is usually one year from the filling date. If you take expensive drugs on an as-needed basis, ask the pharmacist to note the manufacturer's expiration date for you as well. It will often give you extra time as long as you store the medicine properly. While you're talking, ask your pharmacist if he or she knows about any programs in your community that can help you pay for medicines you need if cost concerns you.
- Generic medicines cost less than brand-name medicines and are chemical clones. If there is no generic version of your medicine available, talk with your HCP and pharmacist to see if there is a less expensive alternative medicine that will treat the same condition even if it isn't the identical drug.
- You may be able to save money by shopping for price and get-

ting different medicines at different pharmacies. If you do, you need to take responsibility for checking on interactions since your medicines won't be coming from the same place. You can go to the library and use one of the online drug interaction services, or write down all of your drugs and ask a pharmacist to check them for interactions for you.

- You can cut your drug costs in half in some cases by splitting pills. For eligible medicines, ask your HCP about prescribing a tablet double your usual dose so you can buy a pill splitter (less than $10) and cut them in half. This strategy, however, will not work for every medicine! First, it must be a plain pill without a special coating, and it can't be a capsule. It can't be a time-released drug, and you can't do this with medicines for which precise dosing is critical, like anticoagulants. You'll need the manual dexterity to do this, or have someone who can do it for you; some pharmacies will provide the service for a fee. As long as you understand that pills do not split precisely in half, with careful drug selection and monitoring by the HCP and pharmacist, this can be a viable alternative for patients who would otherwise not be able to afford certain medicines.

- A significant change in medicines in recent years is the shift to one-pill-a-day dosing rather than one pill three or four times a day. While it is easier and more convenient to take just one pill a day, in many cases you can save a lot of money by asking your HCP about switching to a medicine with a less convenient schedule. You have to be sure you will remember to take more than one dose a day, or the decrease in effectiveness of your treatment may wind up costing you more than what you'll save by switching medicines.

- Every pharmaceutical company has a plan of some sort for people who can't afford their medicines. But it is a very complex network that differs from company to company and often within a single pharmaceutical company. The request needs to

## Medicines

| BRAND NAME | GENERIC NAME | DOSE (mg) | TIMES PER DAY | WHEN | FOR WHAT CONDITION | PRESCRIBER |
|---|---|---|---|---|---|---|
| | | | | | | |
| | | | | | | |
| | | | | | | |
| | | | | | | |
| | | | | | | |
| | | | | | | |
| | | | | | | |
| | | | | | | |
| | | | | | | |

## General Health Information

Patient Name_____

Pharmacy Name and Phone_____

Primary Care Provider and Phone_____

Drug Allergies (Name of drug and type of reaction)

_____

_____

_____

Additional Health Information

_____

_____

_____

_____

_____

-------------------------------------------------------------------

Photocopy this form, fill it out, and carry it with you in case you need urgent care. You may also share it with your HCP if more than one person prescribes for you.

go through a HCP or social worker and the medicines are usually delivered to the office—not directly to you. Here are Web sites that will help you learn what programs exist for which medications and the information needed in order for your HCP to make the request on your behalf:

- helpingpatients.org
- rxhope.com (RxHope, 254 Mountain Avenue, Building B, Suite 200, Hackettstown, NJ 07840 Telephone: 1-908-850-8004
- rxassist.org
- needymeds.com

Another resource is the Pharmaceutical Research and Manufacturers of America, 1100 15th Street N. W., Washington, DC 20005, 1-202-835-3400. Your local chapter of AARP should have information as well. (Remember, you can join AARP when you turn 50 for only $12.50. You don't have to be retired.) My advice is to ask a nurse to be your advocate; we know how the system works and I've almost always been successful when I've contacted a company on behalf of a patient.

## LISTEN UP!

Prescription medicines are prescribed for you in a dose that is appropriate for your age, weight, medical condition, and with consideration of other medicines you may be taking. Sharing is a good quality, but *not* for prescriptions. Your prescription should not be open for community use. It might even be dangerous to another family member!

# OTC (NONPRESCRIPTION) MEDICATIONS

## NURSE'S NOTE

The most important thing to do before you buy OTC medicine is to read the Drug Facts label on the back of the package. It may sound obvious, but most people don't! A product can call itself "Pat's Cold and Flu," but that doesn't tell you what the pill, liquid, or lozenge contains. The new labeling system put in place in 2002 makes it easy for consumers because the information has to be listed the same way on every package, regardless of manufacturer, and non-technical language must be used to make it easier for people to understand and compare products.

If you don't read the Drug Facts label carefully, you can get yourself in trouble. A report in the *American Journal of Nursing* described a college student who had a terrible cold. She took different medicines over a few days to treat her different symptoms, including:

- Tylenol to lower her fever
- Cold & Flu Tablets for her "cold"
- Severe Allergy Tablets for her nasal congestion
- Sinus Pain Formula for her facial sinus pressure
- Nighttime Liquid Medicine to help her sleep

What she didn't realize was that every single medicine she took had acetaminophen in it, and four of the five medicines she took contained an antihistamine. She ended up at the student health center drowsy, confused, and disoriented from too much antihistamine, and with early signs of liver toxicity from an accidental overdose of acetaminophen!

If you take your cues from the Drug Facts label, not from the name of the remedy on the front of the box, then you'll be safe. The new format label illustrated here is designed to be similar to the Nutrition Facts label on foods. Herbal remedies do not have a Drug Facts label because they are considered to be food supplements, not drugs. This is an effort by the FDA to standardize consumer information so you can easily find the information you need to make appropriate choices for yourself and your family. Let's go through the parts of the Drug Facts label by reviewing this one from a medicine called Mucinex.

■ **Active ingredient:** This section tells you what's in the remedy you're considering. Each active ingredient is the chemical compound that works in your body to relieve your symptoms. It is

---

# Drug Facts

**Active ingredient (in each extended-release tablet)**      ***Purpose***
Guaifenesin 600 mg.................................................................Expectorant

**Uses** helps loosen phlegm (mucus) and thin bronchial secretions to rid the bronchial passageways of bothersome mucus and make coughs more productive

## Warnings
**Do not use** ■ for children under 12 years of age

**Ask a doctor before use if you have**
■ persistent or chronic cough such as occurs with smoking, asthma, chronic bronchitis, or emphysema
■ cough accompanied by too much phlegm (mucus)

**Stop use and ask a doctor if** ■ cough lasts more than 7 days, comes back, or occurs with fever, rash, or persistent headache. These could be signs of a serious illness.

**If pregnant or breast-feeding,** ask a health professional before use.
**Keep out of reach of children.** In case of overdose, get medical help or contact a Poison Control Center right away.

## Directions
■ do not crush, chew, or break tablet
■ take with a full glass of water
■ this product can be administered without regard for the timing of meals
■ adults and children 12 years of age and over: one or two tablets every 12 hours. Do not exceed 4 tablets in 24 hours.
■ children under 12 years of age: do not use

## Other information
■ tamper evident: do not use if seal on bottle printed "SEALED for YOUR PROTECTION" is broken or missing
■ store between 20-25°C (68-77°F)
■ see bottom of bottle for lot code and expiration date

**Inactive ingredients** carbomer 934P, NF; FD&C blue #1 aluminum lake; hypromellose, USP; magnesium stearate, NF; microcrystalline cellulose, NF; sodium starch glycolate, NF

always the first thing on the label. This label clearly indicates there is 600 mg of guaifenesin in each extended-release tablet. This information is critical since a recommended dose may be one or more tablets. It can get more confusing when you are looking at a liquid product. Be sure you understand how much of each active ingredient (in milligrams or mg) you'll be taking if you follow the recommended dose, listed further down the label under Directions (see p. 102).

■ **Purpose:** This describes the category into which the active ingredient fits. In this case, guaifenesin is an expectorant; in other words, it loosens mucus. Other purposes you may see on different labels include antihistamine, pain reliever, antacid, laxative, and fever reducer, to name just a few.

■ **Uses:** This replaces the more technical term "indications" that you'll see on prescription drug package inserts. On OTC packages, the term "uses" describes the symptoms or diseases the product will treat or prevent.

■ **Warnings:** This part of the label tells you when you should not use (or stop using) the product; under what conditions you should consult your health care provider; possible side effects; age limits; potential drug, food, or alcohol interactions; and how the drug may affect you if you have any conditions such as glaucoma, high blood pressure, asthma, and the like. It will also list any activities you may need to limit while taking a drug, such as not driving if a drug will make you drowsy.

Virtually all OTC labels recommend that pregnant women or those who are breastfeeding consult with their health care provider before use and direct consumers to "get Medical help" or contact Poison Control in the case of an overdose.

■ **Directions:** This section tells you how much you can take, how to take it, how often you can take a dose, and usually the maximum dose in 24 hours. Other important information may be included in this section. For example, for Mucinex, the label states "do not crush, chew or break tablet." This section may also tell you if you need to take the medicine with food or on an empty stomach, or if you can take it without regard to meals. Be sure you don't exceed the maximum dose listed. Pay special attention to this maximum dosing if you are taking more than one OTC medicine, so you don't take an unintentional overdose because two remedies contain the same active ingredient.

▪ **Other information:** This part of the label gives the manufacturer the opportunity to tell you about other safe use aspects of this product that may not fit under another heading. These aspects may include the best way to store the medicine, a description of the tamper-evident packaging used, and the location of the expiration date and lot code on the packaging.

▪ **Inactive ingredients:** These are components of the medicine that do not have a therapeutic effect, but are now listed so that people who have allergies to some of these ingredients will know what is present in a particular product. Commonly, this section will list the colors, flavors, preservatives, and the binders or substances required to hold together a pill or tablet, or the components of a capsule's coating.

## TECHNICALLY SPEAKING . . .

OTC medicines generally treat symptoms, not the underlying problem, so they are designed for short-term use unless under the direction of your HCP. OTC medicines can mask a serious condition and there are time limits on their use. Generally speaking, call your HCP before using these drugs for longer than indicated below.

| OTC GROUP | LIMIT USE TO | REASON |
|---|---|---|
| Antidiarrheal | 48 hours | Risk of dehydration; need to determine cause |
| Antihistamine/ Decongestant | 1 week | Prescription may be more appropriate |
| Constipation | 2 to 3 times per week | Danger of laxative dependence; need to determine cause |

| OTC GROUP | LIMIT USE TO | REASON |
|---|---|---|
| Fever reducer | 3 days | Need to check the source of fever |
| Pain medicine (daily) | 7 to 10 days | Need to check source of pain |
| Skin remedies for rash | 1 week | Need to check for underlying infection |
| Sleep medicines | 1 to 2 weeks | Need to find out why you can't sleep and address cause |
| Sore throat remedies | 2 to 3 days | May need a throat culture to check for strep |

## NURSE'S WISDOM

When you get prescription medicines, safeguards are built in. Access to the drug is limited to people who have a prescription from their HCP, a pharmacist dispenses the drug and checks for interactions, and there is a limit on the amount of medicine you get. When it comes to OTC medicines, the safeguards are your responsibility.

### Storing and taking medicines:

■ The *worst* place to store medicine is in the medicine cabinet in the bathroom. Changes in the bathroom's humidity and temperature will cause medication to break down quickly. Store medicines in a cool, dry place. I use the linen closet in the upstairs hallway, which doesn't get direct sun.

■ If a medicine requires refrigeration, keep it chilled, but make sure it doesn't freeze. If it does, call the pharmacist to see if it is still safe to use once it thaws.

■ Do you have to take a liquid medicine that tastes awful? The colder it is, the less you'll notice the taste.

■ Do you have trouble swallowing pills? A spoonful of applesauce or yogurt helps the medicine go down, and if you momentarily slip any pill in just before you swallow, it won't affect the medicine.

## Drug safety.

You may think that because you can buy OTC medicines without a prescription, they can't be dangerous. Many people regularly take more than the label recommends because they believe their symptoms are worse than those of the average person taking the medicine. I have just one word for you—wrong! Adults who unintentionally overdosed on acetaminophen and had resulting liver damage took a median dose of 5 grams per day; the recommended maximum is 4 grams a day. The difference? Two extra-strength (500 mg) tablets.

Read labels carefully. Of the people with liver damage related to acetaminophen, 25% had taken combination drugs, not realizing how much acetaminophen they were taking. You may not realize that strong prescription pain medicines can also contain acetaminophen, including Lortab, Percocet, Tylox, and Vicodin. To prevent problems when taking OTC medicines, consider the following safety tips:

- Clarify any instructions about taking medicines. Don't assume or guess when your health and safety are at stake!
- Never, ever take medicine in the dark. You could grab the wrong bottle and take the wrong medicine in the wrong dose.
- Don't keep bottles of pills that can change your alertness or judgment next to your bed. You could easily overdose because you can forget how much you've taken. (This warning applies to pain medicine, tranquilizers, sleeping pills, or other sedatives.)
- Don't buy OTC medicines if the package is damaged; that's the purpose of tamper-evident packaging. Bring it to the pharmacist so it's off the shelves.
- Don't take any medicine that looks odd, is discolored, has an odor, or is otherwise different in any way.
- Remember that there is no such thing as a childproof cap or packaging.
- If children don't live in your home (and you haven't made your

home child safe), be particularly vigilant if kids come to visit, or if you travel with medicines to a place where children will be present (holidays are a particularly risky time). Make sure medicines are put away in a place the children can't get to—not in a pocketbook, open suitcase, or the guest bathroom vanity.

■ Never use silverware to measure a teaspoon of liquid medicine. Most people are surprised to learn there is no standard size for silverware teaspoons. They can range from a half teaspoon to two teaspoons in fluid measurement. Instead, do what we do in the hospital: switch your thinking to milliliters or mL (the same thing as cc's) and get a syringe from your HCP or pharmacy.

| | |
|---|---|
| 2.5 mL | = ½ teaspoon |
| 5 mL | = 1 teaspoon |
| 15 mL | = 1 tablespoon |
| 30 mL | = 1 ounce |

Ask your favorite nurse to show you how to measure liquid medicine using a syringe and how to draw up different amounts by mL so you'll always be accurate.

■ Make sure every professional prescribing for you knows all the medicines you take, including OTC, herbal remedies and nutritional supplements. Don't withhold information from anyone prescribing for you, particularly if you have not been taking medicine as prescribed. If there is no clinical improvement, better to have a talk with your HCP about why you haven't been taking the medicine than to make him or her waste time trying to figure out why the medicine (you're not taking) is not working.

■ Ask if there are any blood tests you need while taking a prescription drug—either to measure the level of the drug in your blood or to measure the drug's effect on your body. If you need blood tests, don't skip them; they are critical to make sure your dose isn't too high or too low and you're not developing complications.

■ Keep your medicine in its original container—particularly if you are traveling. You never want to wonder what pill you're taking! If in doubt, throw it out.

■ If you are taking a drug that will sedate you, such as an antihistamine, pain medicine, or tranquilizer, let someone in the household know.

■ Discard old medicine, medicine you don't take anymore, and medicines that have given you bad side effects. There isn't consensus on the best way to discard medicines. The American Association of Poison Control Centers recommends flushing medicines down the toilet, but there have been reports of floating pills at water treatment centers because they didn't break down. Never put them in the trash where children or animals could get hold of the medicines. Check with your local pharmacy to see if they have a program that lets you drop off discarded medicines. Me? I put medicine through my garbage disposal with plenty of water so the medicine is chopped up, diluted, and flushed away.

## Interactions.

When you choose a new OTC medicine, find out if there are any interactions with food or other medicines you're taking. Interactions work many ways. Consider two drugs that interact. For example, Drug 1 (Maalox, OTC for heartburn) may block the absorption of Drug 2 (metroprolol, a prescription drug that controls heart rate and blood pressure), thus decreasing the level of Drug 2 in your blood. You may wind up with higher blood pressure or an irregular heartbeat—in other words, the symptoms you're taking the metroprolol to control. Or the interaction of Drug 3 (ibuprofen, OTC anti-inflammatory) and Drug 4 (warfarin sodium, or Coumadin, a blood thinner) will greatly increase the blood-thinning effects of both medicines, perhaps to the point of putting you in danger of internal bleeding. To prevent interactions, consider the following:

- Be responsible for checking for interactions because you are essentially "prescribing" the OTC medicines for yourself. Often, there won't be signs of an interaction until you have trouble on your hands. For example, you won't have any symptoms if interactions decrease the effectiveness of birth control pills or high blood pressure medicine, but there could be substantial consequences down the road.
- Compile a list of your medicines (prescription, OTC, and herbal) and then compare them on a web site to see if there are interactions among any of the remedies in the group. Three web sites to try are drugdigest.org, drugs.com, or drugstore.com.

## ALPHABETICAL LIST OF INGREDIENTS AND USES

With all the OTC medications available, it's easy to mistakenly buy two different medications containing active ingredients that actually do the same thing, or one containing an ingredient that treats symptoms you don't have.

This list organizes common OTC drugs alphabetically and includes their specific use. My hope is that you will take this book into the pharmacy. When you consider a remedy, you can take the package off the shelf and use this list to check the ingredients to make sure you are getting what you need to treat your symptoms—and no extra medicine for problems you don't have.

There are far too many drugs to cover them all, but the list that follows includes ingredients found in the most popular OTC drugs. If you have any questions, be sure and ask the pharmacist before you make your purchase, or check with your HCP.

| DRUG NAME (GENERIC) | USED TO TREAT |
| --- | --- |
| Acetaminophen | Pain, fever |
| Acetaminophen/Aspirin/Caffeine | Migraine pain |
| Aluminum salts | Indigestion/heartburn |
| Antazoline phosphate with naphazoline | Eye irritation or allergies |

| DRUG NAME (GENERIC) | USED TO TREAT |
| --- | --- |
| Aspirin | Fever or pain |
| Aspirin/Caffeine | Pain |
| Attapulgite | Diarrhea |
| | |
| Bacitracin | Skin injuries or conditions |
| Benzocaine | Mouth or skin pain |
| Benzocaine/Menthol | Sore throat |
| Bisacodyl | Constipation |
| Bismuth subsalicylate | Indigestion/heartburn/diarrhea |
| Brompheniramine maleate | Allergy symptoms |
| Butoconazole nitrate | Vaginal yeast infection |
| | |
| Calamine | Skin irritation/itching |
| Calcium as antacid | Indigestion/heartburn |
| Camphor/Lidocaine | Mouth pain or irritation |
| Castor oil | Constipation |
| Chlorpheniramine maleate | Allergy symptoms |
| Cimetidine | Indigestion/heartburn |
| Clemastine fumarate | Allergy symptoms |
| Clotrimazole | Fungal infections more commonly known as "athlete's foot" and "jock itch" on the skin, thrush in the mouth, and vaginal yeast infections |
| | |
| Dexbrompheniramine maleate | Allergy symptoms |
| Dextromethorphan | Cough suppressant |
| Dimenhydrinate | Motion sickness |
| Diphenhydramine hydrochloride | Allergy symptoms |
| Docosanol | Mouth pain or irritation |
| Docusate | Constipation |
| Doxylamine succinate | Allergy symptoms |
| Dyclonine hydrochloride | Sore throat |
| | |
| Famotidine | Indigestion/heartburn |

| DRUG NAME (GENERIC) | USED TO TREAT |
|---|---|
| Glycerin (rectal) | Constipation |
| Guaifenesin | Cough—loosens mucus |
| Hydrocortisone topical | Skin irritation/inflammation |
| Ibuprofen | Pain, fever |
| Kaolin with pectin | Diarrhea |
| Ketoconazole | Fungal infections more commonly known as athlete's foot and "jock itch" on the skin |
| Ketoprofen | Pain |
| Loperamide hydrochloride | Diarrhea |
| Loratadine | Allergy symptoms |
| Magnesium citrate | Constipation |
| Magnesium hydroxide | Indigestion and heartburn; constipation |
| Magnesium sulfate | Constipation |
| Methylcellulose | Constipation |
| Miconazole | Vaginal yeast infections |
| Mineral oil/petrolatum/shark liver oil | Hemmorrhoids, rectal itching/irritation |
| Naproxen | Pain, fever |
| Neomycin/polymyxin B/bacitracin | Skin injuries or conditions |
| Nicotine | Smoking withdrawal symptoms |
| Nizatidine | Indigestion/heartburn |
| Omeprazole | Indigestion/heartburn |
| Oxymetazoline nasal | Stuffy nose |
| Oxymetazoline ophthalmic | Eye irritation, redness |
| Pheniramine maleate with naphazoline | Eye irritation, redness |
| Phenol | Sore throat |
| Phenylephrine | Hemorrhoids, rectal itching/irritation |

| DRUG NAME (GENERIC) | USED TO TREAT |
| --- | --- |
| Phenylephrine hydrochloride | Stuffy nose |
| Pramoxine hydrochloride | Hemorrhoids, rectal itching/irritation |
| Pseudoephedrine | Stuffy nose |
| Psyllium | Constipation |
| Ranitidine | Indigestion/heartburn |
| | |
| Senna | Constipation |
| Simethicone | Intestinal gas, bloating |
| Sodium bicarbonate | Indigestion/heartburn |
| Sodium phosphate | Constipation |
| | |
| Ticonazole | Vaginal yeast infection |
| Tolnaftate | Fungal infections more commonly known as "athlete's foot" and "jock itch" on the skin |
| Triprolidine hydrochloride | Allergy symptoms |
| | |
| Undecylenic acid | Fungal infections more commonly known as "athlete's foot" and "jock itch" on the skin |
| | |
| Witch hazel | Hemorrhoids, rectal irritation/itching |
| | |
| Zinc sulfate ophthalmic | Eye irritation, redness |

## LISTEN UP!

Taking one pill is not necessarily better than taking three different pills. A single combination pill containing an ingredient you don't need is worse than taking three different pills that specifically target your symptoms. This is particularly true when treating colds, flu, sinus symptoms, and allergies. In our home, we have single-ingredient drugs so we can take only what we need.

Single-ingredient products also give you more control over dosing. If, for example, you have high blood pressure, you may want to take a smaller dose of decongestant to reduce the potential side effect of elevated blood pressure. But if all you have is a multisymptom pill, you'll have to take the full dose of each ingredient whether you need it or not.

Finally, remember your OTC and prescription medicines in your emergency preparedness plans. Be sure you get your medicines at least seven to ten days before you'll run out and think through what you would do if you didn't have power or running water for a few days. You may want to keep a few days' supply at your workplace and/or at a friend's or relative's home in case you can't get back home right away. Ask your pharmacist about whether you can store your medicines in your car or if the temperature extremes would affect your particular drugs.

## IS IT A MEDICATION ALLERGY OR A SIDE EFFECT?

### NURSE'S NOTE

I became aware of this common confusion when, in one shift, three patients told me they "were allergic" to different medications. When I asked, "What happened when you took the medicine?," here's what patients told me:

- "I'm allergic to amoxicillin. I got a yeast infection when I took it for strep throat."
- "I'm allergic to codeine. It made me sick to my stomach and woozy."
- I'm allergic to Benadryl because it made me very sleepy."

Feeling sick to your stomach or woozy isn't fun (we won't even talk about yeast infections), but these are side effects, *not* allergic reactions. An allergic reaction can be life-threatening and needs to be dealt with immediately. For side effects, there is a much wider variety of signs and symptoms to bother you.

Why is confusing allergies and side effects a problem? Let's say a woman believes she is allergic to amoxicillin because she got a vaginal yeast infection while taking amoxicillin for strep throat years ago. If she writes down amoxicillin when asked about drug allergies, she will not be treated with any antibiotic from the penicillin family, even if one of those drugs is the best for an infection she has now. That's because no HCP wants to get sued for giving someone a medicine the medical record says she is allergic to, even if the medical record isn't correct!

Self-diagnosed "allergies" like this limit the medications from which the HCP can choose and potentially pose serious risk to your health.

## GET THEE TO THE ER

Call 911 for a trip to the ER if, while taking a medication, you:

- Develop hives.
- Develop red skin on most parts of your body.
- Have unexplained itching all over after taking the medicine, particularly on your scalp and on the palms of your hands.
- Develop swelling of the lips, tongue, or eyelids.
- Feel a lump in the throat or have trouble swallowing.
- Have trouble breathing, with or without wheezing.
- Feel chest tightness.
- Feel palpitations, or an irregular or very fast heart beat.
- Get woozy or lightheaded.
- Develop a cough that sounds like croup, or like a seal barking. If not controlled, this kind of allergic reaction can cause swelling that will close off your airway so you won't be able to breathe. This is a major emergency, and not a situation in which you should go to the ER on your own unless you are a

block away. You need the expertise of emergency medical service professionals for this trip.

If you know you have an allergy, and have had an exposure or possible exposure to a medicine to which you know you're allergic, go to the ER if you have the slightest indication of the signs and symptoms listed above. These early signs of an allergic reaction can progress even more rapidly if you've had a reaction in the past.

## CALL YOUR HEALTH CARE PROVIDER

- If you do not have a known allergy, and you notice a rash (usually red and blotchy), hives, or itching and *no other symptoms*.
- If you're experiencing a side effect that's troublesome, such as a bad headache that interferes with your daily activities. You may need to try different drugs to find one that strikes the balance of minimal side effects while providing effective treatment.
- If you want to stop taking a medication because of side effects, such as a headache or constipation. Managing side effects is all about teamwork with your HCP. Get in touch with the prescriber, talk about what you're feeling and explore your options.

## TECHNICALLY SPEAKING . . .

During an allergic reaction, your immune system, which is supposed to fight off foreign invaders such as bacteria, viruses, and other potentially harmful substances, goes overboard. The immune system mistakenly identifies a medication that's supposed to help as something harmful that the body must fight against. Medications that commonly trigger allergic reactions include:

- Penicillin (and related drugs such as amoxicillin)
- Sulfa antibiotics (such as sulfamethoxazole, a component of Bactrim and Septra)

- Allopurinol (used to treat gout)
- Some blood pressure medications.
- Some antiseizure medicines such as phentytoin (Dilantin) and carbamazepine (Tegretol)

However, anyone can have a reaction to any medication. And it doesn't have to be the first time you take a drug; sometimes it takes multiple doses for the immune system to mount a full-blown reaction. Unfortunately, there is no reasoning with your immune system to explain it has made a mistake and get it to back off.

As opposed to an allergy, a *side effect* is a secondary effect you experience while taking a drug that is not the intended therapeutic action of the drug. Many side effects are a nuisance, but they are not as potentially harmful as a full-blown allergic reaction.

It's important to be aware of any major side effects that could affect your everyday functioning, such as becoming drowsy if you take an OTC antihistamine like diphenhydramine, which is also found in OTC sleeping pills. You don't want to take one of these pills before you have to drive or, as the warning label says, "operate heavy machinery." You also need to know if you should avoid drinking alcohol or taking other medications that could interact with the one you're taking. (For example, aspirin can enhance the blood thinning effects of the anticoagulant Coumadin.)

Common side effects include:

- Being drowsy (occurs with many OTC antihistamines, medicines with "PM" or "night" in their names, prescription pain medicine)
- Feeling jittery, hyperactive, or unable to settle down enough to fall asleep (common with decongestants and too much caffeine, which is in some OTC pain medicines)
- Feeling sick to your stomach, or not feeling like eating
- Cramps and diarrhea (particularly with antibiotics)
- Constipation
- Feeling lightheaded

**❓ Frequently Asked Questions**

Q. *What's the difference between a side effect and an adverse effect?*
A. In the practical world, they are the same thing. If you read medical literature, you're more likely to see the term "adverse effect."

Q. *My father is allergic to penicillin. Does that mean I will be?*
A. There is no evidence that drug allergies are inherited or run in families.

Q. *What should I do if I am having a side effect?*
A. The best thing is to call the HCP who prescribed the medication or recommended an OTC drug for you. If you are having a side effect from an OTC drug you chose on your own, simply stop taking it. If it is a prescription drug, what you'll do depends on how severe the side effect is; that is, does it prevent you from going to work or school, or carrying out your daily activities? If that's the case, you'll need to stop taking the medicine and talk with your HCP about a suitable alternative. Or the side effect may be uncomfortable, but you can live with it (such as a headache) to see if it goes away over time because there isn't a good alternative drug for you to take. This is all very individualized; the best approach is to have a talk with your HCP.

■ Headache, which usually goes away after a week or two if it occurs when you begin a new medicine prescribed for you to take daily on a long-term basis

## NURSE'S WISDOM

■ In my home, when one of us gets a new medication, the other reads the side effects. The "patient" then starts the medication. If something changes—for example, I get a dry mouth or headache—my husband checks the side effects to see if those changes can be attributed to the new medication.

- Side effects may happen one time and not at another since they depend on a number of factors, such as other medicines you're taking at the same time—particularly OTC drugs or herbal remedies you might not think about—and your diet, stress level, and even amount of sleep you did or didn't get.

- Get to know your local pharmacist, even if your insurance requires you to buy most of your prescriptions through the mail. Your community pharmacist is a wealth of information, just a phone call away and often available when the HCP's office is closed or the mail-order pharmacist has gone home.

## SELF-CARE

- If you have a true drug allergy, remind your prescriber whenever you're handed a new prescription for anything—even eye or ear drops. Ask, "This is OK even though I'm allergic to penicillin, right?"

- If you have a true drug allergy, get an ID bracelet and wear it all the time. I've nearly died from allergic reactions to drugs twice and have a Medic-Alert bracelet on my ankle, where it's out of my way, but will still be seen by medical personnel if I'm unconscious. (Call 1-800-ID-Alert to get yours.)

- When you get a new prescription filled, ask if there is anything you should do to reduce side effects, such as taking medicine with a meal, on an empty stomach, at bedtime (if the drug will make you drowsy), or in the morning (if the drug is likely to make you a little hyper).

- Don't look for trouble. If you are waiting for a side effect to occur, it probably will!

- If you take prescription medicine every day, check with the pharmacist before choosing an OTC remedy for self-treatment of another condition to reduce the risk of side effects for each drug when you take them both in the same day.

■ Resist the urge to treat a side effect with another drug unless you've had a long talk about your options with your HCP.

## LISTEN UP!

If you think you are having a mild allergic reaction, talk to your HCP or, if it's the weekend and no one is readily available, stop in and see your community pharmacist. A trained professional will know what an allergic rash looks like, the characteristic description of symptoms, and what drugs are and are not likely to cause allergic reactions. Do not decide on your own that you're allergic; eliminating a drug or class of drugs from your care could have serious repercussions in the future.

The next time you fill out a medical history form, if you did have a reaction, describe it when you write down drug names under "allergies." For example: "Penicillin: rash, trouble breathing, throat almost closed; Keflex: hives."

# ANTIBIOTIC ALERT

## NURSE'S NOTE

One hundred years ago, infections were the leading cause of death in the United States. Not anymore. Antibiotics are truly wonder drugs. But you shouldn't wonder about whether antibiotics are right for you. Work with your HCP and understand that if you have a common viral infection, what you really need is time, sleep, and some hot chicken soup—not antibiotics.

Many HCPs admit that they often write antibiotic prescriptions to satisfy their patients—more as a customer service than good medical practice. For example, about 21% of all antibiotic prescriptions—about 2.5 million—are written for patients with colds and bronchitis when there is no solid evidence of bacterial infection—

just to keep patients happy. Instead of demanding that prescription, start a dialog with your primary care provider to discuss if antibiotics are appropriate for your illness.

## INSIDER INFO

Antibiotics are medicines used to treat bacterial infections. There are different types of antibiotics because there are so many different strains of bacteria that can cause illness. Prescribing antibiotics requires a thorough understanding of which bacteria are likely to cause a particular type of infection, and which antibiotic is most likely to kill those bacteria. For example, a throat infection and a bladder infection are usually caused by very different bacteria, and the antibiotic that would be best for your urinary symptoms won't work as well (if at all) for your sore throat.

Over the years, bacteria have become more difficult for antibiotics to kill. Bacteria can quickly change their cell structures to fend off antibiotics. This is a particular problem if you don't take all the pills in an antibiotic prescription. Naturally, you'll begin to feel better quickly. Then most people either forget to take pills, or stop taking them intentionally because they think the infection is gone. Usually, the weakest bacteria are killed first. But when pills are not taken long enough, the heartier bacteria survive. Not only do they survive, but since they have "seen" the antibiotic, they can change their structure so that the antibiotic will not kill them in the future. It's similar to the way a coach can change his game plan for the second half of a game after studying the opponent during the first half. When this happens, the bacteria are said to be "resistent" to a particular antibiotic.

If you don't take all the pills in your antibiotic bottle, you may still get better. But you can infect someone else, and the common antibiotic you took may not kill the slightly changed bacteria in other people. Another, more expensive antibiotic with more side effects may be required. The concern in the health care community is that the back-up antibiotics are not as effective as they once were, and

---

**?** **Frequently Asked Questions**

Q. *How can my HCP tell if I have a bacterial infection?*

A. A test called a culture should be done to determine which bacteria, if any, are responsible for your illness. A companion test, the sensitivity test, then determines which antibiotics are most effective against that particular organism. More and more experts strongly recommend that a culture and sensitivity test be done for *every* patient before antibiotics are prescribed, which means no more antibiotics over the phone. And you should ask for the culture and sensitivity test if your HCP does not suggest it before prescribing.

---

there are fewer back-ups to choose from. Eventually, there may be "super bugs" that no antibiotic will kill.

## TECHINCALLY SPEAKING . . .

The Alliance for the Prudent Use of Antibiotics lists 15 different categories of antibiotics with multiple drugs in each category. Choosing the appropriate antibiotic before culture and sensitivity results are back is the art and science of clinical practice. There are two general categories: *broad-spectrum* antibiotics stop the growth of many different bacteria, and *narrow-spectrum* antibiotics only work against specific organisms.

Antibiotics can't be targeted precisely to kill only bacteria causing your Strep throat or your pneumonia or the Staph infection in your skin. The drugs will also kill off beneficial bacteria in your body, particularly those in your intestine and, in women, those in the vagina that keep yeast in check. Losing beneficial intestinal bacteria can result in diarrhea, bloating, and gas, and losing normal vaginal bacteria can allow a yeast overgrowth, otherwise known as a yeast infection.

## NURSE'S WISDOM

- Resist the convenience of having antibiotics prescribed over the phone without an exam.
- Ask your HCP about a culture and sensitivity test before you start taking antibiotics.
- If antibiotics are prescribed, follow the instructions on the bottle exactly. If the pills are prescribed for three or four times a day, try to space them evenly throughout the day while you're awake.
- Keep taking the antibiotic until the prescription is finished, regardless of how soon you feel better.
- If you take birth control pills, ask if the antibiotics will make the contraceptive less effective.
- Ask the pharmacist whether you should take the pills with meals or on an empty stomach, or if it matters.
- Ask if you should avoid any foods while taking the antibiotic—for example, you should avoid consuming dairy products and taking antacids within two hours of taking an antibiotic from the tetracycline family or the common antibiotic Cipro (ciprofloxacin).

## LISTEN UP!

The smartest approach is to talk with your HCP about whether you should have antibiotics instead of demanding a prescription when you are sick.

# HERBAL REMEDIES AND NUTRITIONAL SUPPLEMENTS

## NURSE'S NOTE

Herbal remedies and nutritional supplements are becoming more popular every year. But choosing a product is fraught with challenges for the consumer. Since I would need a whole book to discuss everything you should know about herbal remedies and nutritional supplements, in this section, I'll give you tips for making your choices, things you need to be careful about, and resources I use for reliable information about complimentary therapies.

When it comes to herbal remedies and nutritional supplements, many people trained in the traditional medical model pale. First off, many of us were taught that we direct care and the patient is on the receiving end. These complimentary therapies are almost all consumer driven, thus throwing off the old balance of the doctor as the single prescriber who controls what you take.

And, here's another little secret: most HCPs know little or nothing about complementary medicines because formal education hasn't caught up with the explosive product growth in this area. When you've been trained in a traditional approach to health care that is based on pharmaceuticals, as I was, it's hard to shift gears, and can be even harder to find reliable information so we can be as up to date and comfortable discussing herbal remedy options as discussing traditional pharmaceutical options. And it's critical to remember that herbal remedies are drugs and should be respected as such.

The challenge is separating the science from the charlatans.

## GET THEE TO THE ER

Herbal remedies and nutritional supplements behave in the body in much the same way traditional pharmaceuticals do, with almost none of the safeguards that exist for pharmaceuticals. That means you can have allergic reactions, serious side effects, and complications from taking these products, just as you can with pharmaceuticals.

Call 911 for a trip to the ER if you have any serious change in your condition as you would after taking any pharmaceutical.

## CALL YOUR HEALTH CARE PROVIDER

Check in with your HCP before taking any herbal remedies or nutritional supplements if:

■ You take any daily medicines (prescriptions or OTC).

■ You have any chronic illnesses such as asthma, diabetes, heart disease, high blood pressure, HIV, and the like, or if you're being treated for cancer.

■ You are pregnant or trying to get pregnant.

■ You have any questions or concerns about whether a particular remedy is right for you.

## INSIDER INFO

It's hard to know where to start, so instead of covering the variety of supplements available, I'll give you information about how the industry is regulated and what you should look for in order to be a wise consumer.

### The role of the FDA.

Most important, know the FDA's role in overseeing herbs, vitamins, minerals, and other dietary supplements is *not* under the "drug" umbrella, but rather the "food" side of the agency. That alone should be a huge red flag that snaps you back to reality when your eyes glaze over from all the choices on the shelves in the stores today. Regulation comes from the Dietary Supplement Health and Education Act (DSHEA) that was signed into law in 1994. Under this law, a company that puts products in the market is responsible for determining that its supplements are safe, and that any claims are substantiated by evidence. This means these products do not need or receive FDA approval before they go on the shelf. In fact, unless it is a new dietary ingredient, a company does not even have to provide the FDA with the evidence it relies on to back up its safety or effectiveness claims (it's supposed to keep the information on file in case the claims are ever challenged).

Companies do not need to register with the FDA, nor are there regulations that establish minimum standards for manufacturing dietary supplements. In general, they are the same standards in place for foods.

**Labeling requirements.**

The FDA has minimum labeling requirements that include the following:

- Descriptive name of the product, clearly stating it is a dietary supplement.
- Name and place of business of the manufacturer, packer, or distributor (including contact information if the consumer wants or needs additional information).
- Complete list of both active and inactive ingredients.
- Net contents of the product (such as the number of capsules or ounces of liquid).

There must also be a Supplement Facts panel similar to the Drug Facts on OTC drugs (see p. 213) and the Nutrition Facts label on foods. This section must include every dietary ingredient contained in the product, how much of the ingredient is in each "serving" (such as one capsule or tablet), and the "other ingredients" listed in order from the ingredient in the highest amount to the lowest (as "other ingredients" are listed on a food label).

**What else you'll see on a label.**

This is a marketing world, and when I looked on the shelves of my local pharmacy, I did not see a single herbal remedy or nutritional supplement that did not have what's officially called a structure/function claim. This is where you need to be cagey. You see, if a label said a product could treat, prevent, or cure a specific disease or condition, then it would be an unapproved—meaning illegal—drug. Since no one wants an illegal product in their store or warehouse, very careful language is used instead. The FDA published a list of "Approved Health Claims" for foods that will keep the company using the claim out of trouble. Here's a comparison between food and supplement claims labeling:

- My oatmeal box says, "Three grams of soluble fiber daily from oatmeal in a diet low in saturated fat and cholesterol may reduce the risk of heart disease. This cereal has one gram per serving." This is an approved health claim.

■ By contrast, my bottle of echinacea says, "Echinacea may help stimulate natural resistance by helping maintain the immune system. Echinacea is very popular because it's used to

---

## Frequently Asked Questions

Q. *Since herbal supplements aren't considered drugs, I don't need to tell my doctor about them, right? I don't want him to make fun of me.*

A. If you are afraid to be up front with your doctor, or any HCP ridicules you, you need a new HCP (see p. 243). Putting that issue aside, even though these products are classified as dietary supplements in the United States, substances such as echinacea, St. John's wort, garlic, ginseng, and ginkgo are used as drugs in much of the rest of the world. They can interact with traditional pharmaceuticals—for example, ginkgo and aspirin both reduce blood clotting, so you shouldn't use them together, and St. John's wort can make some birth control pills less effective. You should tell your HCP and your dentist if you take any OTC medicines or nutritional supplements regularly, and they should go on your personal drug list just like prescription medicines.

Q. *Can it hurt to try an herbal supplement? If they're "all natural," they must be safe, right?*

A. Anthrax spores are found in soil, and soil is natural. Does that convince you that the word "natural" has nothing to do with "safe"? There is no official definition of the word "natural" as it applies to supplements, and no rules about standards of manufacturing purity or safety that must be met before the word "natural" is put on a label. And, yes, it can hurt to just try supplements because there is also no rule requiring manufacturers to list side effects as drug manufactures do. I can't emphasize this point more strongly. You need to respect that herbal medicines can cause serious side effects and drug interactions, just like traditional pharmaceuticals can.

strengthen and enhance overall health and well-being. American Indians used Echinacea—also called Purple Coneflower—during the winter season." This is followed by: "These statements have not been evaluated by the Food and Drug Administration. This product is not intended to diagnose, treat, cure or prevent any disease. . . ." (This is a structure/function claim, used because only a drug can treat, cure, or prevent diseases and this is a *dietary supplement*).

You'll also see directions on the label for how many pills or drops of a liquid to take how often, but again, those are not approved by any external regulating organization or agency. It is up to the com-

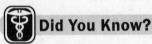 **Did You Know?**

*Harris Interactive Health Care News* reported in October 2002 on a nationwide survey conducted on anti-aging medicine, vitamins, minerals, and food supplements. Here are key statements tested, and the results:

- "The government requires that [supplement] labels include warnings about potential side effects or dangers."
  *68% said this was true.*
- "Supplements must be approved by a government agency like the FDA, which approves pharmaceuticals before they can be sold to the public."
  *59% said this was true.*
- "[Supplement] manufacturers are not allowed to make claims for safety unless there is solid scientific evidence to support them."
  *55% said this was true.*

Actually, *none* of these statements is true. Clearly, we need to supplement consumers' knowledge before they buy dietary supplement products.

pany to have the data on file that substantiate their structure/function claim and their directions for use.

## NURSE'S WISDOM

- Just because someone is behind the counter at a store in which nutritional supplements and herbal remedies are sold doesn't mean they know anything about the products. Least harmful is a clerk who doesn't know anything and just tries to be helpful; worst is the sales clerk who gets a financial bonus for selling certain products. Unless you are in a pharmacy and know you are talking with the pharmacist, be very, very careful about who is giving you advice.

- Herbal remedies and nutritional supplements are popular in multilevel marketing programs. You may trust a friend or acquaintance who gives you a presentation about a special supplement powder she mixes into a healthful shake every morning, but what makes her an expert on your health?

- No herbal remedy or nutritional supplement needs to be bought immediately; if you are getting pressured to buy a product, walk away.

- Read labels carefully; it can be hard to match up a reputable reference book with what you find on the shelf. Particularly when you're looking at herbal remedies, there are tinctures, capsules, tablets, powders to mix with water, creams, gels, and lotions, and it can be difficult to figure out if the reference's dosage recommendations are accurate for the form you're considering.

- Supplements and herbal remedies are not a substitute for a reasonable diet that includes a variety of foods.

- Seek out information about side effects; you're not likely to see any mentioned on a label.

- Never replace a pharmaceutical with an herbal remedy without checking with a qualified professional first.

- If it sounds too good to be true, it is. If you don't get enough sleep, a supplement such as caffeine will help keep you going for a day or two, but the bottom line is that you need the sleep, and there is no supplement to make up for that.

## LISTEN UP!

Who are you going to get advice from when considering an herbal remedy? I got lucky and struck up a conversation with a local community pharmacist who had done a fellowship in botany and herbal medicines, and he was knowledgeable, objective, and helpful. If you are in a store and getting advice from someone, ask what their background and qualifications are. Fortunately, more and more schools of pharmacy are offering courses in botany and herbal medicines.

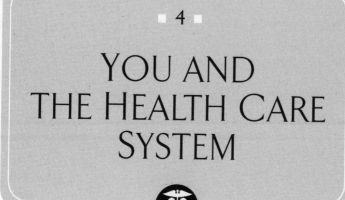

**4**

# YOU AND THE HEALTH CARE SYSTEM

# CHOOSING YOUR PRIMARY CARE PROVIDER

## NURSE'S NOTE

Choosing your primary care provider (PCP) is one of the most important decisions you'll ever make. Your PCP should be your advocate, working with you to help you manage symptoms, illnesses, injuries, or any conditions you have. Your PCP should also be available by appointment when you are sick, and by phone within 24 hours when you have a question (or today, maybe by e-mail).

As nurses, we usually have "the skinny" on who's good and who's not. And don't you buy that line, "If Dr. So-and-So is on the staff, he must be good." There are doctors who could charm the bark off a tree, but that doesn't mean they know what they're doing medically. On the other hand, most nurses can tell you about the cranky doctors they'd call for in an emergency because they are such skilled, knowledgeable practitioners (and not for their bedside manner). You've hit pay dirt when your PCP is pleasant, warm, engaging, *and* on top of his or her game clinically.

## Choosing a new primary care provider.

People have different hot buttons when it comes to choosing a PCP (who can be a physician or nurse practitioner). Some prefer a woman; others don't care. You may have geographic preferences. Sometimes the age of the provider is a factor. Here's a list of factors for you to consider. Only you can decide which are and are not important, and their priority. If any of these are "deal breakers," do your homework beforehand, either on the Internet or by making phone calls and getting that critical information as a way to narrow the list of candidates you'll interview.

- Do you have a preference whether your PCP is a physician or a nurse practitioner? How do you feel about a practice in which you may be seen sometimes by the doctor and sometimes by the nurse?
- Does your health insurance policy have requirements that you use a provider from an approved list in order for your visits to be covered? That may limit your options.
- Is there a particular hospital you would prefer to go to? Is your hospital choice limited by your insurance plan? If so, then you'll need a PCP affiliated with the specified hospital(s).
- Do you feel strongly about having a man or a woman as your PCP?
- Is the age of your PCP important? Would you feel comfortable with a PCP younger than you? Are you looking for a long-term relationship? Some people prefer older providers who have a lot of experience; other people prefer younger providers who may be more technologically savvy and have recently finished the rigors of training.
- If you've settled in an area and plan to spend a long time there, you may want to think about establishing a relationship with a PCP whose age is close to yours or a little younger—not a PCP who is three or four years from retirement.
- Is it important to you that your PCP went to school in the United States? The number of physicians and nurses coming to

the United States from overseas schools continues to rise, so the issue is likely to come up when you are considering a new PCP. I have known great doctors who went to medical school outside the United States, and lousy doctors with great pedigrees from top U.S. schools. It's your call; if you feel strongly one way or the other, check it out in advance.

■ If you're considering a nurse practitioner as your PCP, he or she will be board certified. If you are considering a physician and he or she is not, find out why. Board certification is an outside verification of the practitioner's knowledge beyond the licensing examination. It's designed for consumers. You may decide you won't consider a physician who is not board certified, or you could make it one of your interview questions. A terrific community-based family practitioner may simply be too busy to make arrangements for time off to sit for the boards.

■ Do you have strong feelings about your PCP's specialty?

■ Is the office location important? Would you prefer that it be nearer your home or your workplace? Are you willing (or able) to travel some distance if you find a special PCP with whom you can have a great relationship? Or, do you need someone nearby?

■ Are there limits on hours you could see your PCP for routine care, such as a physical or checkup because of your work schedule, for example, or can you be flexible? If office hours are an issue for you, check in advance before you make that interview appointment.

■ Are there any providers in the area you would not want caring for you under any circumstances? If so, before you make an interview appointment, ask what doctors or practices cover the off hours for the provider you're considering. You may be switching providers because of a bad experience, and find out later that your new doctor shares "on call" responsibilities with the one you left and never wanted to see again! Check it out.

## Frequently Asked Questions

**Q.** *Should I choose a provider in internal medicine or family practice as my PCP?*

**A.** Which one you choose is entirely up to you, unless there is some unusual restriction from your insurance company. Specialists in internal medicine limit their practice to caring for adults, while those in family practice can care for the entire family (and you'll often share the waiting room with sick kids). Some people like the idea of "one-stop shopping" for the whole family, while others prefer a little more separation and privacy. Young adults, in particular, may prefer to finally be away from a waiting room with toy blocks and *Highlights* magazine.

**Q.** *What is board certification? Is it part of being licensed?*

**A.** Board certification is a level above licensure, in which doctors and nurses take "state board" exams that assess a baseline level of knowledge needed to practice safely upon graduation from school. Licensure does not involve specialty knowledge. Technically, the initials "RN" represent the professional titles that come with licensure and tell you nothing about an academic degree. "MD" is the degree awarded by the medical school; an MD may never be licensed to practice medicine if his or her work is in the research laboratory. An RN is always licensed; an MD usually is, but you should check to make sure.

Both nurses and doctors can be board certified. They can take examinations in their respective specialty areas if they meet certain educational and experience requirements. If they pass the exam(s), they're board certified.

**Q.** *Is it important to have a board-certified care provider?*

**A.** It depends. While board certification is technically voluntary (unlike licensure, which is mandatory to provide patient care), few physicians entering practice these days will forego certification. For nurses (except nurse practitioners), board certification remains totally voluntary. Thus, board-certified nurses are a special group who have taken the extra step to validate their knowledge and make a long-term commitment to professional excellence.

Many health care organizations make board certification a requirement for their medical staffs. However, less than half of family practice doctors are board certified, so there are clearly well-qualified doctors out there who simply haven't taken the exam. This may be because they are based in communities more often than hospitals or academic centers where board certification is required for faculty or staff appointments. An umbrella organization, the American Board of Medical Specialties (ABMS), coordinates activities for 24 medical specialty boards. You can call them at 1-866-ASK-ABMS (275-2267) to verify an individual physician's credential(s).

Q. What's the difference between a nurse and a nurse practitioner?

A. A nurse practitioner is also called an "advanced practice registered nurse." These nurses have additional education beyond their basic nursing school, and have a special license that allows them to practice more independently than nurses who are not qualified for advanced practice. Each state has its own law about the drugs a nurse practitioner can prescribe and how their practice is supervised. Nurse practitioners can specialize in many areas such as pediatrics, family medicine, or even critical care.

■ Do you have strong beliefs that would affect your comfort level with a particular provider? For example, would you be comfortable or uncomfortable if you knew that a physician you are considering performed abortions, or would it be immaterial?

Once you've narrowed it down, confirm that the provider you are interested in is accepting new patients. Make an appointment to interview the candidates who have the opportunity to be your PCP. Yes, *you* interview *them*. Some may think you're crazy, but then maybe those are the folks you don't want to work with. Ask for a meet-and-greet appointment first, but if the front-office people won't give you one, then make whatever appointment they want you to make—such as a physical or regular office visit. Then you can control the agenda for the visit once you're there.

## INSIDER INFO

### How I found a new PCP.

I had been with the same PCP for about 15 years and knew him since we worked together in his first year out of medical school. About four or five years ago, the practice started to become more troublesome than helpful. It was nearly impossible to talk to a human when I called the office. Messages went unanswered for days at a time, and half the time they got lost.

That should have clued me in that it might be time to make a change. Still, I hung in there because of my long-term relationship with my doctor (as you may be tempted to do). Then, I got a "Dear Patient" letter from the doctor telling me he was no longer going to provide primary care because his specialty became too busy. It was time to move on.

I decided to ask friends and other doctors for recommendations and the feedback led me to an internal medicine group at a local university medical center. You may or may not be comfortable receiving your care at a practice affiliated with a medical center and medical school. Doctors and nurse practitioners who practice in this setting tend to be interested in teaching medical and nursing students and learning new things themselves, and they are often members of the faculty. If you have chronic health conditions, a medical center may be most convenient for you, and it may be best if you have an unusual diagnosis. Since I remember what it was like to be a student, I don't mind being examined by a student. You may feel differently, however, and may prefer to choose a practice that is not as involved in the educational process.

I called the office to make an interview appointment, and ended up talking with one of the office assistants. I asked if she knew any of the doctors in internal medicine. She said, "Oh, Dr. Manger is the nicest man. I'm sure he's a good doctor, but I like him best because he's always so polite and really nice to work with." Bingo. A doctor who treated the office staff well? Sounded like my kind of guy.

After a ten-minute chat with the doctor, I knew I had found a good match for me. How did I know? Because when I told him I was looking for a PCP who would be my partner in my health care, he replied, "That's great. I much prefer to work with patients who feel that way." We then had a discussion about philosophies of care, and his obvious knowledge of medicine coupled with respect for the fact that I was an expert about *me* sealed the deal.

### Lessons learned:

1. Never put up with a miserably run practice because you feel a sense of loyalty. Many of us overlook problems with the practice and office staff that really make things far more difficult for us as patients because of our relationship with the doctor. Tell the doctor about the problems you're having and how they make things more difficult for you, give it a few months, and if there is no response or change evident, move on.

2. In my experience, the nurses and doctors who treat those lower on the totem pole with the same respect they show to colleagues or superiors are the ones you want to hook up with. When the woman who answered the phone at the doctor's office said Dr. Manger was nice to her, I was reasonably sure I'd found my new PCP, and I was right.

### Evaluating your relationship with your PCP.

Like any successful relationship, the one you have with your PCP needs attention and fine-tuning. Here are key factors to regularly reevaluate to make sure you've got the right provider for your needs:

- Are you pleased with the relationship overall? Is your general sense one of being satisfied or dissatisfied? If you're satisfied, great. If you're dissatisfied, hopefully the following points will help you clarify what the problem is.

■ What's your gut feeling about the office staff? Do they grate on your nerves or are they pleasant and treat you with courtesy and respect? If you have a problem with someone, get his or her name and be sure to tell your PCP. The people working "in back" examining and treating patients often have no clue how the front desk, telephone, and waiting room are handled.

■ Have you developed a rapport with your PCP? In plain terms, are you comfortable with your PCP's approach to you, approach to the practice, and for lack of a better term, "bedside manner"?

■ Is your PCP willing to sit and talk with you, or do you find yourself talking faster and forgetting what you really wanted to ask because the PCP stands with one hand on the doorknob, waiting to leave? Routine talk time should be built into your appointment. If you feel like you're on an assembly line, get five or six minutes with your PCP, and then you're whisked out of the exam room so they can get the next person in, *speak up*. If you need to have a lengthy discussion, for example about the pros and cons of surgery for a condition you have or about whether hormone replacement therapy is right for you, ask about making a separate appointment just to talk.

■ Do you have any concerns about your PCP's competence or fitness to practice?

■ Do you feel like you can be totally honest with your PCP, or do you hide things? Are you reluctant to be candid (about smoking or alcohol use, for example) because you don't want to hear a lecture? Are you afraid you might be ridiculed or treated differently? Is it because the PCP treats other members of your family, or you know that the clerk who answers the phone and has access to records is a blabbermouth? Then find another PCP.

■ Finally, beyond the customer service and personality issues, do you trust your PCP? Do you trust her and the staff to maintain confidentiality? Do you trust him to make referrals or order tests based on what's in your best interest, not because he has a financial incentive in the deal? Do you trust her to commit to lifelong learning and to keep abreast of new research and clinical practice guidelines so you are getting the most appropriate care?

These are issues that most people don't think about specifically; it's more of a gut feeling that something's not right. Hopefully, these questions will either reassure you that you've got a good match, or help you identify what isn't working. Then it's up to you to decide if you need to move on, if you think you need to call Dr. Phil for help saving the relationship, or if you can work it out with a talk on your own.

## LISTEN UP!

- You are the boss when it comes to your health.
- You have the right to ask for second opinions and change health care providers if you are not satisfied with the care you are receiving.
- Don't turn to mush when you deal with a physician. As one who has worked with thousands of doctors over the years, I can assure you that M.D. does *not* stand for "major deity." They're people just like you and me. If you are afraid to say something to your doctor, ask yourself if you would feel the same way if you were dealing with your auto mechanic or plumber. You "hire" the physician. If you're not treated with respect, or no one returns phone calls, or you can't get an appointment, it's time to go elsewhere.

# GETTING THE MOST FROM YOUR RELATIONSHIP WITH YOUR HEALTH CARE PROVIDERS

## NURSE'S NOTE

I can't emphasize enough that in today's health care environment, you need to think about assembling your own all-star team. To continue the sports metaphor, you are the general manager and your PCP is your coach who can help recruit, oversee, and coordinate the work of other team members.

For many years in our culture, the doctors "called the shots." But we are moving to a more collaborative approach to care that focuses on the patient and in which doctors, nurses, pharmacists, and other professionals are all contributing members of the team. This approach is better for everybody.

## Members of your health care team:

- **The general manager.** That's you—the one who hires and fires and puts the team together. You will have ideas from the skybox—a big-picture view of how reasonable a given treatment plan is considering your day-to-day responsibilities. For example, if your PCP recommends physical therapy for your bursitis, but the physical therapy office hours are the same hours you have to take care of your mother, it's your job to say, "That may not work, and here's why." Dialogue and collaboration are the keys to success. It's your job to speak up and provide feedback to your PCP. Otherwise your PCP won't be able to get the most out of the team for you.
- **The coach.** That's your PCP. He or she will have ideas from the

field level, knowing the condition, the optimal treatment, and all the things you *should* do.

It's important that your PCP doesn't eliminate your right to make choices. For example, you are having lower back pain and your PCP says, "Let me refer you to a neurosurgeon." If you want to see a chiropractor first, you should be able to make that call. And your PCP should be willing to work with a chiropractor and prescribe medication if necessary. You shouldn't be forced to choose between one (the traditional medical model) or the other (the chiropractic physician).

On the other hand, if you've selected carefully, your PCP's point of view usually has merit. You may be convinced you need to see a chiropractor, but if your PCP can tick off five reasons chiropractic care won't help your condition, he or she might have a point.

- **The team.** Seeing specialists when necessary gives you a diverse team for all-star care. For example, a woman will want to include an OB-GYN. A man who regularly plays golf may want to include an athletic trainer who can help with specific exercises to prevent muscle strains and sprains. If you have asthma, a respiratory therapist can help teach you how to manage your symptoms to minimize flare-ups.

## INSIDER INFO

### When you make an appointment:

- Plan your time depending on how you keep track of appointments, how punctual you are, and what you know about the PCP's likelihood of being on schedule. It never hurts to make a quick call before you leave for the appointment to see if they're running behind. If you're tight on time and can leave 20 minutes later rather than sitting in the waiting room cooling your heels, everyone's happier.
- Ask in advance if you will need blood work (For example, if you're having a physical). If you need blood work that's best

done on an empty stomach (for example, for glucose and cholesterol tests), ask for the first appointment of the day. Why starve till an 11 a.m. appointment if you don't have to?

- If you don't need to fast or have tests, ask the office staff for the inside scoop about what appointment times are best—for example, when the office is less busy, when the PCP is less likely to run late, or when the PCP doesn't have to run out for a committee meeting. I am not a morning person, so I usually shoot for the first appointment after the office lunch hour; if the morning was running late, the break gives them catch-up time.

- Getting the run-around from the office person who controls the phone? Ask to leave a message on the doctor's voicemail. If they won't put you through or you know the doctor rarely checks voicemail, wait until they turn the phones over to the answering service at the end of the day, and then ask the answering service to page the doctor you need to talk to.

## How to get the most from an office visit:

- Find out what you should bring to the office with you. If you take any medicines every day, particularly if they are from different prescribers, many HCPs will want you to bring *all* your medicines in their original bottles to each visit so they can be sure not to prescribe a new medicine that would interact.

- Bring a crib sheet. It might be a list of questions for your PCP, or aspects of your family medical history you wanted to share, or the name of a prescription renewal you need. In fact, I'm disappointed when I don't see patients bring notes. I'm afraid they'll remember something they wanted to ask when they're halfway home.

- Don't take on the burden of diagnosing yourself. Remember Sgt. Joe Friday of *Dragnet* and report "Just the facts, ma'am." Instead of announcing to your PCP, "I have an awful sinus infection," try it this way. "For the past three days I've noticed increased congestion in my nose. In fact, I have to breathe through my mouth it's so bad. I'm having trouble sleeping and I'm coughing up green stuff. Oh, yes, and I also have a miserable headache." Let your PCP put it together; he may think of something that didn't automatically jump to your mind. Then, you can discuss the approach—together.

■ If you don't want a particular piece of information written in your medical record, such as a history of childhood sexual abuse or a history of drug abuse (but you've been clean for 15 years and your family doesn't know) but you want your PCP to know about it, tell him there is something you would like to discuss. Add that before you disclose it, however, you want to know if he will keep it out of the record. Unless it's something that must be reported by law, there's no rule that says every single thing has to go in your record—particularly if you can explain why you don't want it committed to paper.

■ If you see a specialist or receive care from any other professionals, ask them to send a letter to your PCP describing your care. Have copies of any test results sent to your PCP. Ideally, your PCP should be the repository for your most complete medical record.

■ What is the office routine for patient calls? Some PCPs, particularly those in family practice who deal with Mom questions, have special telephone hours during which they take calls directly. If your PCP's practice isn't set up that way, find out the best way to leave a message, whether you can speak to another member of the office staff or whether there is one nurse or assistant who always works with your PCP with whom you can establish a relationship.

■ Is your PCP willing to correspond on e-mail? This is great for quick questions if you check your e-mail at least once a day. E-mail can also eliminate phone tag. Although you need to be judicious about how much personal information you write or receive in an e-mail, if your e-mail is password protected, it may provide you with more privacy than if you got a phone call or message left on the family answering machine. Be aware, however, with the HIPAA regulations—government orders about patient privacy that went into effect in mid-2003—some HCPs will not correspond this way for fear of breaching privacy.

## LISTEN UP!

If your relationships with health care providers have been ones in which you usually sit passively and do whatever the doctor tells you without asking questions, you may want to reconsider. Don't let that examination gown turn your resolve to mush.

There is so much you can gain by being an active participant in your care. You can explore alternatives rather than settling for whatever the doctor says. You can build a relationship with your HCP in which there is an ongoing dialog. If you have a way to get your questions answered in a reasonable period of time, whether by telephone or e-mail, you can address small issues whenever they arise—before they become big problems. You may want to try a visit with a nurse practitioner; nurses can offer a different perspective on your care that you may find refreshing.

# INSURANCE SCRABBLE: MAKING SENSE OF THE LETTERS

## NURSE'S NOTE

Trying to decipher the abbreviations and codes used to describe health insurance plans today can be as confusing as trying to figure out what police officers and firefighters are saying when you listen in on a scanner. Is that a 10-4 on your 10-20?

In today's health care world, you need to understand how the system works so you can make the best choices for yourself and your family. I'll give you an insurance-to-English translation and a road map to follow that will help you end your journey, if not in the Heavenly Health Care Penthouse, at least on the first floor of the building. I'll be your tour guide because I've navigated this route when making these choices for my family, and I have seen firsthand the wrong turns many of my patients have unknowingly taken. Your thoughts about the choices you made on the insurance forms when everyone in the family was healthy may change abruptly if a surgeon says the word "cancer" is in your new diagnosis.

## INSIDER INFO

When managed care was moving into the marketplace in the 1990s, there were initially aggressive incentives to hold costs down. The scary parts for the patient were two particular approaches: profit sharing and information control.

In profit sharing, the physician's income was directly tied to the resources used by the patients. That is, if patients didn't see a lot of specialists, or have a lot of tests, or take expensive medicines, costs were held down and the physician would get a nice cash bonus. This raised questions in some patients' minds about whether their doctor was making decisions in their best interest or in the best interest of his wallet.

Information control was a process by which physicians were actually muzzled by insurance companies. They were not allowed to present the entire range of options to patients with complex conditions; they could only talk about those covered by the insurance plan.

Once these little secrets became public, there was a huge uproar. HCPs can now talk about anything with patients, and fewer physicians get bonuses for keeping costs down by limiting patients' access to care. However, that doesn't mean you should keep your head in the sand as a consumer.

## TECHNICALLY SPEAKING . . .

MCOs, PPOs, HMOs—what's the difference? Following are the technical definitions of all those insurance acronyms. Keep in mind, though, there are many hybrids. Use these as a starting point for deciphering the options your employer offers or those you find on your own if you're self-employed or not covered by a company plan.

## MCO (Managed Care Organization).

This broad term describes a plan, insurance company or group of health care providers that focus on controlling costs while providing quality care. This is primarily accomplished by controlling patient access to the health care system and reviewing and evaluating whether services requested are appropriate and necessary.

Patient access is controlled through lists of "participating health care providers" and requiring patients to choose their providers from this list. Otherwise, insurance won't pay. These health care providers have agreed to provide their services at a discount to the MCO. These lists can be a real problem when you change insurance plans either because your company got a better deal with a different company, or you changed jobs. If you're lucky, you can keep seeing the same health care providers. If not, when your insurance changes, so do all your doctors, nurses, and practitioners. You can imagine how annoying that can be and that things can fall through the cracks when transferring your care to a different practice.

MCOs also control access by making it inconvenient for you to see a specialist, whose care is more costly. Many plans require you to obtain a written referral from your primary care provider before you can see a specialist. If the primary care office staff is efficient, the referrals won't be too much trouble. If they're not efficient, you can spend a lot time trying to get them to send the right form to the right specialist at the right time so you can keep your appointment.

The tight control on access to services has eased some in recent years. After consumer complaints that MCOs were depriving members of needed health care, most states instituted independent review boards and rapid appeals programs. These boards give patients and their health care providers the chance for prompt reconsideration of a claim.

## HMO (Health Maintenance Organization).

Many people use this term to describe all types of MCOs, but they're not the same. HMOs are the granddaddy of the MCOs. The first was started by Henry Kaiser, a California entrepreneur, in the 1930s. He contracted with groups of physicians to provide health care services to his employees and even built company-owned hospitals and clinics before health insurance for workers was commonplace. HMOs were originally designed with these features:

- A purchaser (employer or insurance company) buys a health care service package from health care providers and hospitals for a prepaid, monthly fee.
- The premium is paid regardless of the amount and type of services provided.
- The HMO owns the facilities and employs the health care professionals that members must use for their health care needs. Members cannot go outside the system unless they want to pay for the outside care themselves.
- Physicians are typically paid a salary plus an incentive bonus if costs are kept down and the HMO makes a profit.

The benefit to the employer and consumer is the fixed cost so they can budget for the year knowing exactly what health care costs will be. The HMO takes all the financial risk. The consumer's choices are severely limited to those offered by the HMO unless they are willing to foot the whole bill themselves.

In the 1990s, a number of hybrids of this original HMO model became more popular, focusing on contracting with physicians in private practice. The basic principles are the same, however: needed care is provided for a fixed monthly fee.

Because health care costs are climbing again, more costs are being shifted to the consumer. This is one reason you need to be savvy. It is also why pure HMOs are not as common today; they cannot afford to shoulder the financial risk.

### PPO (Preferred Provider Organization).

PPOs were designed to address concerns about the restrictions that come with a traditional HMO. In a PPO, independent practices sign a contract to provide services to plan members at discounted rates. Practices get less money, but most are forced to join or they won't have any patients.

If a patient selects a preferred provider (one who is contracted with the plan) the patient is rewarded by paying less for services, usually in the form of a "co-pay." If the patient chooses to receive care from a provider outside the plan, the patient will have to pay more, but not the whole cost as in an HMO. These plans are more expensive for patients, as more of the financial risk shifts from the MCO to the consumer. The benefit is that consumers have more options to choose the health care providers they want to see and the facilities where they want to receive care.

### FFS (Fee-for-Service).

This is the system many of us grew up with. There were no lists. You went to any health care provider you liked, sent the bill in, and the insurance company paid it. These are also sometimes called "indemnity plans." The providers received a fee for each service provided.

The problem was that there were no cost controls, and health care providers had an incentive to do more procedures and run up the bill. A few FFS policies are out there, but as you can imagine, they are very expensive. My prediction is that before long this type of insurance will be seen only in a health care museum. You can go there and regale the grandkids with stories of . . . the good old days.

If you have a choice among plans or coverage options, set aside a day or a long evening with your records from last year and a calculator. Tally up what you paid for your health care last year. Here's how you can figure it out:

| Family member | Harry age 32 | Ruth age 28 | Jackee age 3 |
|---|---|---|---|
| Primary care visits | 0 | 3 | 5 |
| Specialist visits | 0 | 2 | 1 |
| One-time prescriptions | 0 | 3 | 7 |
| Daily prescription meds | 0 | 3 | 0 |
| Dental care | Cleanings | Cleanings | Routine |
| Planned surgery? | Yes, bone spur | No | Maybe ear tubes |
| Pregnancy? | No | Yes, due 6 mos. | No |

**Frequently Asked Questions**

Q. *So, which type of insurance plan is best?*

A. "Best" depends on your personal circumstances. If you're just out of college, single, have no health problems, no HCP preference, and need coverage in case you break your ankle or need to have your appendix removed, the "best" plan for you will probably be the most restrictive, least expensive plan for starters. On the other hand, if you have a chronic condition like asthma, for example, and you have a great relationship with your HCP, your "best" plan is the one that lets you continue to see that HCP and covers your medications without a lot of money out of pocket over and above your premiums.

Many people, especially new moms, like more structured health plans, particularly those that provide no-charge access to telephone advice nurses. It's a great way to have simple questions answered, and a real treat if you have ever left a message at your HCP's office and then sat around all day waiting for a return call while you wondered if your child was really ill or not.

In this example, Harry has no chronic health conditions, but he has a bone spur in his heel for which he's put off surgery for a year. Ruth has asthma, for which she takes daily medicine and sees a specialist. She's also currently four months pregnant with their second child. Jackee, their daughter, had four ear infections in the past year, and she may need to have tubes inserted in her ears for drainage.

When you take the time to see just how much you spent in the previous year, you will be better able to predict expenses in the coming year. Check your options paying special attention to the following:

■ Is there a deductible (out of your pocket before insurance kicks in), and if so, how much?
■ How much will it cost you for each visit to your primary HCP?
■ How much will it cost you for each visit to your specialist(s)?

- How much is the co-pay for each one-time prescription at the local pharmacy?
- How much is the co-pay for each daily medicine refill? Is there a price break by using mail order and getting a 90-day supply? (If so, that will mean four co-pays for a year of refills). Is there a formulary (a list of preferred medicines) that assigns different prices to different drugs? If so, calculate the cost from your pocket for each medicine for the year.
- Then, look through the plan specifics for the reimbursements that cover your anticipated needs in the coming year. In this example, it will be outpatient surgery, prenatal care and delivery, and well-baby care, but don't forget blood tests, X rays, and the like.

Add up your out-of-pocket costs under the different plans offered. Then, multiply your contribution per pay period by the number of pay periods you have in a year to determine your total deduction for the plan.

Out-of-pocket #1 + Payroll deduction #1 = Your estimated total health costs for option #1

Out-of-pocket #2 + Payroll deduction #2 = Your estimated total health costs for option #2

Finally, think about the intangibles that are important to you, such as does one plan require referrals, does another require a change of HCP? Convenience and choice may be worth paying $100 or more extra a year.

Also, when you are checking out a health plan, be sure you understand your access to emergency care. At one time, insurance companies refused to pay for claims if the discharge diagnosis didn't indicate an emergency, regardless of the symptoms that brought the patient to the ER. We had patients sitting at home with chest pain because they weren't sure it was their heart, and if the heart tests turned out negative, their insurance wouldn't pay, because, in retrospect, it was not an emergency. Now, if patients have a reasonable concern that their symptoms are due to a very serious condition, the insurance companies are supposed to pay according to the initial symptoms, not the final diagnosis. Still, it may take a few phone calls and letters to get things straightened out.

Some insurance plans require approval for a visit to the ER unless it is a true life-threatening situation no one would argue with. When you sign in, the clerks in the ER check your coverage, and if needed, they'll call to get an approval code for your visit. If the company says no, it's up to you whether to stay, but you'll have to sign a form that you were informed the visit will not be covered by your insurance.

Other plans may require that you call an advice line—usually staffed by registered nurses—before going to the ER for all but the most serious conditions. The nurse will discuss your symptoms with you, and based on standard treatment protocols, advise you whether to go to the ER or to wait for an office visit later in the day or the next day. Of course, you always have the right to go to the ER at any time for any reason, but if you don't follow your insurance plan's rules, they may not have to pay, leaving you stuck with the bill.

## LISTEN UP!

Let's face it, health insurance can be terribly confusing, and if you feel like you can't get a straight answer from anyone, you may be right. Here's the problem; your employer probably won't be able to answer specific questions about plans because it will not assume the responsibility for interpreting the fine print from the insurance company. Expect your benefits department to be very hands off during the decision period. And, the insurance company may not be much help either because it's hard for them to justify spending money on customer service representatives for potential customers who are kicking the tires. But, don't give up without a fight. Get your questions answered before signing on the dotted line. Your decision now will have an impact on your care for the next 12 months.

# TIPS FOR ER VISITS

## NURSE'S NOTE

Having, um, let's just say more than 20 years' experience, I have seen the incredible changes in our health care system from my ring-side place at the bedside. (In the ER, of course, I rarely found time to have a ringside *seat* to anything!)

One thing I know for sure is that the changes have not all been to your benefit. That's why I want to share this insider's guide so you can team up with the nurses and work the system in your favor.

## INSIDER INFO

There's a huge nursing shortage, and it's not going to let up anytime soon. Nurses are being stretched to the limit, and we are incredibly frustrated that we have less time to spend with our patients even to just hold a hand and talk since touch and rapport are such impor-tant aspects of healing.

Fortunately for me, I haven't had to be an ER patient all alone in the past 20 years. If there is anyway you can bring someone with you, I strongly recommend it. If you're really sick, you'll need some-one with a clear head to get you there (and probably back home) and to get instructions and look out for you in general so there is less you have to think about.

As I stated before, it's an unwritten ER rule that any female be-tween the ages of 10 and 70 is pregnant unless proven otherwise. Don't be offended if your nurse asks more than once or if four dif-ferent people ask, "Any chance you're pregnant?" or "When was your last menstrual period?" as you're getting ready to go to X ray. Likewise, Mom, don't be horrified that a pregnancy test is being done on your 16-year-old daughter. If I had a nickel for every teenaged girl who swore she's never had sex and turned out to be pregnant, I'd have enough money for a condo in the Virgin Islands.

Another inside tip: every ER has a blanket warmer, which is a warming cabinet that *should* be kept full of blankets. They're there in case someone comes in with a very low temperature (as can happen if you're in a car crash in the rain and come in soaking wet). But, if you just plain don't feel good, a warm blanket can be dreamy. Wrap it tightly around your body and cover it with a plain blanket to hold in the heat. If you're a patient, or with a friend or loved one, ask for "a blanket from the blanket warmer, please." When I'd begin my shift, the first thing I'd do was check to see that the blanket warmer was full. I may not have been able to spend a lot of time with my patients, but offering one cozy, warm blanket spoke volumes.

## NURSE'S WISDOM

### Bring a relative or friend along.

A "care partner" can watch your belongings if you have to go to another part of the hospital (for an X ray, for example). He or she can keep you company to help the time pass and can follow up with the nursing staff if you've been waiting for pain medicine or test results. Particularly when you feel really miserable, it's awfully nice for you to be able to sleep and let your care partner do the thinking for you.

Fact is, nurses are completely swamped with work in ERs. Unfortunately, nurses these days have less time (if any!) to spend on the little niceties that may not cure but certainly help a patient feel better, such as placing a cool cloth on your forehead when you're feverish and have a headache or tucking you in with a pile of blankets when you're freezing. If a care partner is with you, he or she can quickly learn where the blankets and pillows are to help meet your comfort needs when we can't be there immediately.

### Feed nothing, starve everything ... unless we say it's okay.

Once you sign in to the ER, don't eat or drink (or give the patient something) unless you've cleared it with the nurse first. It's best to follow this rule from the time you walk in the door, even when you are in the waiting room. Why? Food or drink could delay surgery, interfere with a test result, or interact with medication you may need. When a family member of a patient I'm not working with asks for apple juice for the patient, I say, "Let me check." If the nurse caring for that patient says it's okay for the patient to eat or drink, then I point out the fridge or get the juice for them myself. If I always check, you should, too.

### Ask before you go to the bathroom.

We may need a specimen. Want to see a grown nurse cry? Have him wait for an hour and a half for a patient to urinate, only to walk into the room as he hears the toilet flush. If you don't want to sit around until you can go again, check first. Or, it may not be safe for the patient to be walking or moving around (if there's a chance of falling or being woozy from medication, for example). Always check with the nurse first.

### Bring a list of your medications.

Be sure you don't leave anything out. (see p. 210). We may not be able to administer certain medicines because they could interact with something you're already taking. This is particularly critical with Viagra, which leads me to the next point.

### Tell the truth.

People in the ER have pretty much seen it all. If you don't tell us something or try to hide something from us, the results could be very hazardous to your health. For example, many men are reluctant to say they take Viagra. But if you don't tell us you've taken it, and you are having symptoms of a heart attack, we will usually give you a nitroglycerin-type drug to increase blood flow to your heart. The problem is that when these drugs are combined with Viagra, your blood pressure can plummet. A potential heart attack is bad. A potential heart attack with very low blood pressure is worse than bad. That's just one example of how hiding important facts can be dangerous—and even life-threatening.

Another common issue is how much alcohol you regularly drink (or have consumed that day) and any recreational drugs you use. We don't call the police. But if you lie about the amount of alcohol you've consumed, for example, and you come to the ER because you fell and broke your ankle, the combination of the pain medicine we are likely to give you and the alcohol in your system could make you unconscious. We *really* hate it when that happens.

### Tell the whole truth.

Don't leave out information in your history, such as not telling us if you've HIV positive, or have hepatitis or diabetes. We won't segregate you if you're HIV positive. But if you are HIV positive and have a fever, cough, and chest pain when you take a deep breath, we may need to do different tests for you because you may have a different type of pneumonia than someone who is not HIV positive.

### Ask for privacy if you need it.

If you want to tell us something that you don't want the person you came with to know about, give us a signal of some sort. I've made it a habit to begin my interviews with patients by asking anyone with the patient to step outside the room. That way, we can get any confidential information out of the way. If the patient says, "No, she can stay," and the problem is a simple one such as a cut on the finger, I might not push it. But remember that if you're the patient, you have a right to speak privately to your nurse and any other health care provider.

### Bring something to pass the time.

Obviously, this isn't an issue if you're in really bad shape, but if you feel fine and are in the ER because you don't know if your ankle is sprained or broken, or if you need stitches, or if you're someone's "care partner," bring a magazine or book. I don't go anywhere for an appointment without a couple of issues of *Reader's Digest* tucked in my purse. Distraction beats clock watching, hands down.

### Keep us posted on your condition.

While you're a patient in the ER, it's very important to let us know if your condition changes. If you're given medicine, ask the nurse who gives you the medicine how soon you should feel some relief. If, for example, the medication we've given you hasn't made a dent in your abdominal pain after an hour, be sure to let someone know.

If you have a new symptom, such as numbness on your right side in addition to the headache that made you come to the ER, tell us right away. If we did something that makes you feel better, such as giving you a drug that got rid of your nausea, we want to hear about that, too. If you're feeling better, we can think about sending you home, and if we know which medication helped you, we can more effectively plan for your at-home care.

### Remember, there are no stupid questions.

When leaving the ER with instructions, you *must* understand them. For example, if you've been told you can't put any weight on your injured knee and you're handed a pair of crutches, you'll need to practice with them before you leave. If the nurse doesn't suggest you walk up and down the hall a few times to learn how to use the crutches safely and make sure they fit properly, ask him or her to walk with you and give you feedback about your technique.

You, your ER nurse, and any other health professionals that treat you are all on the same team with the same goal, which is getting you or your loved one better and moved through the system, either by admitting you to the hospital or by sending you home. You have a responsibility to be honest and do the best you can to communicate fully and accurately with your ER nurse. Your ER nurse has the same responsibility to you.

### SELF-CARE

Before you head home from the ER, here's what you need to know:

### Medications:

■ If you are being given any medicine to take home or prescriptions to be filled, review the name of the drug, why it has been prescribed, and whether this is a drug for long- or short-term use.

---

**?  Frequently Asked Questions**

Q. *What's the difference between the ER and the urgent care center?*
A. An ER is for emergencies that threaten life or limb; an urgent care center is like sophisticated doctor's office. It's important to know the options for care in your community. Urgent care centers can be self-contained in a strip mall or near a town center apart from the hospital, or the hospital ER can have a separate section for people who are "office sick," often called the "fast track" because you get in and out much quicker than the regular ER. Urgent care centers have limited hours; even those in the hospital building aren't open 24/7. Most are open into the evening and on weekends and holidays, though. You can always call the urgent care center in your community to check the hours and ask if they can manage your problem. For example, some urgent care centers will put in stitches, some don't. For others, it depends on the location and the nature of the injury and whether you'll need X rays and deep cleaning of the cut.

---

■ Find out if the medicine is for use "as needed" (for pain, for example) or if you should take it on a schedule. If you know how the medicine is supposed to work, you can use it most effectively.

## Okay and not okay symptoms:

■ If you've had an injury, know what symptoms are to be expected and which are signs something's wrong. For example, if you broke your ankle and you're in a cast or a splint, it will hurt. For many people, that pain will be significant and is to be expected. But you don't need to come back to the ER. However, if your toes get cold and blue, that means the blood flow to your foot is reduced, usually because of swelling. You'll need to get back to the ER right away.

■ Ask how you're supposed to feel the next day. For example, if you've been in a relatively minor car crash, you may be shook up, but have no sign of injury when we check you out right after the crash and your adrenalin is in overdrive. However, by the next morning, you may not be able to turn your head because of muscle spasms in your neck (more commonly called whiplash). Knowing what to expect can keep you from panicking. I always told my patients about this because it happened to me when I was in college. The morning after my crash when I couldn't turn my head, I was convinced I had a broken neck. If I'd only been warned, I wouldn't have been terrified about moving.

■ Be sure to get written instructions from the ER that says something like, "If [fill in the blank] happens, come back to the ER."

## Following up with your HCP.

After an ER visit you'll usually be instructed to follow up with your regular HCP. But if the HCP in the ER wants you to see a particular doctor (such as an orthopedic specialist for a broken bone), remember these magic words: "I was seen in the ER last night and they told me I need to see Dr. So and So tomorrow [or in two days, or in one week]." Amazingly, doctors whose schedules are packed for six months will be able to fit you in if the ER says you have to see them for follow-up. (Just promise me you won't use these magic words any time you want an appointment!)

If the doctor's office staff refuses to give you an appointment in the ER suggested time frame, you have a few choices:

■ You can call the ER back, ask for the nurse in charge, and explain that you've been unable to get an appointment. The ER can often call the doctor's office for you, or refer you to another doctor.

■ You can call the hospital's main switchboard and ask for the medical staff office. Part of having hospital privileges is agreeing to see ER patients in referral. If a doctor is refusing, tipping off the medical staff office might just get you in as soon as you're supposed to be seen.

■ Finally, you can call your PCP's office for advice.

## LISTEN UP!

Be sure to follow through with the instructions you receive. Have your stitches removed on the date specified, schedule the ultrasound test, call your health care provider, or follow a special diet—whatever the instructions say. Even if you don't agree with the ER treatment plan, at minimum, follow up with your HCP who knows you best. Then you can be sure nothing falls through the cracks that could make your condition worse.

# TIPS FOR HOSPITAL STAYS

## NURSE'S NOTE

Today, you can't identify the caregivers without a scorecard in most institutions. Just about anyone can wear white uniforms or scrub clothes, and in most cases you can't tell the nurses from the assistants or the housekeepers just by looking at them. One nurse I know wore her old white dress uniform and cap to the hospital as a costume on Halloween, and was shocked when patient after patient told her how much they appreciated seeing a "real nurse."

It might be comical if the potential outcomes weren't so deadly serious. As a health care consumer, it is essential that you know who is taking care of you, whether the care is provided in a regular hospital or another type of facility such as a rehabilitation hospital.

## INSIDER INFO

There can be a huge difference in the care provided by hospitals in the same city or long-term care facilities in the same town. The key to your stay will be the quality of the nursing care you receive. The only way you can be sure you get quality care is by checking on it yourself.

Registered nurses are the key to safe and effective care. When people are admitted to the hospital, they aren't admitted for more "doctoring"; they are admitted for *nursing* care. Intensive care for critically ill patients means intensive *nursing* care. It's the nurse who monitors and checks the patients 24 hours a day. Nurses are the ones who pick up subtle changes in patients' conditions and do whatever is needed to head off complications and help make patients more comfortable. Who's who on the nursing staff? In health-care today, there are basically four levels of nursing personnel:

**1. Registered nurses (RNs)** are generally recognized as the leaders of the bedside health care team. Registered nurses are licensed by each individual state, and basic nursing schools now offer either an associate's degree or a bachelor's degree (nurses can go on to get master's and doctoral degrees, too). Graduates of each degree program take the same exam and receive the same RN license.

RNs are responsible for the overall nursing care a patient receives. The RN is the one who examines and interviews patients, and then designs the nursing plan of care. RNs can provide all the care themselves, or they can select certain aspects of care that they can delegate to other caregivers. The RN is responsible for evaluating the patient's response to the care provided and determining if the plan needs to be changed. RNs are also ultimately responsible for patient teaching—that is, making sure patients understand what they need to know to manage their disease or condition at home themselves or with their family.

**2. Licensed practical nurses (LPNs)** (also called licensed vocational nurses in some parts of the country) traditionally have one year of training in a vocational technical school. They provide patient care, but most state laws require LPNs or LVNs to work under the direction of an RN or physician.

**3. Certified nurse's aides (CNAs)** are workers who take a short course in basic patient care procedures usually taught by an RN.

CNAs assist nurses by helping patients with tasks such as maintaining personal hygiene, taking the vital signs of stable patients, and transporting patients to other areas of the health care facility for treatments, tests, or therapy. CNAs alert nurses to changes in patients' conditions.

**4. Advanced practice registered nurses (APRNs)** are RNs who have had advanced education and training beyond the RN license. Most people recognize these nurses as nurse practitioners, but this category also includes nurse midwives and nurse anesthetists. Each state determines how much these nurses are allowed to do independently. In some states, APRNs can prescribe any medication; in others, the types of medication that can be prescribed is limited. APRNs must pass a special examination in order to receive this advanced license.

**5. Nonregistered nurses and assistants** also work at hospitals and other facilities. The big problem today is that those institutions are receiving less money from insurance companies and the government to pay for the care they provide. As a result, many institutions are replacing nurses with assistive personnel. Make no mistake, these workers are not the nurses' aides who have worked with RNs for years. This new class of worker is trained by each individual hospital. The institution decides what tasks the assistant will perform. There are no standard training programs, no external oversight, and no credentialing. The workers may not even have high school diplomas, yet they could be taking your blood pressure. They can be called nurse techs, patient care technicians, or any other title the hospital chooses.

When hospitals and other health care facilities replace RNs with these assistants, patients may go for hours before a qualified RN has a chance to examine them. Fewer nurses mean fewer opportunities to pick up early, subtle changes in patients' conditions. Caught early, a number of potential problems can be easily taken care of by the RN. Left to simmer, simple problems can become complicated and more difficult to treat.

One aspect of this change in personnel mix that troubles nurses

# MEDICAL TESTS

Having medical tests can be a nerve-racking experience. If you are concerned something is seriously wrong, waiting for results can feel like an eternity. The testing process itself can be inconvenient if you have to take time off work or find a sitter, and it can be even more aggravating if the people doing the tests don't take the time to work with you to reduce any discomfort that may be associated with positioning or any other aspect of the test.

Since I have been around this testing block more than once, I've learned that the better prepared you are before your test, the more accurate your results will be. There's also a lot of flexibility in the system if you'll just speak up. This section will provide you with tips and hints about different types of tests and how to get the best results with the least discomfort.

Let's start this section with the most important tip of all: If your HCP wants to do tests, you should always ask this question, "What will you do differently, or how will my care be affected by the results of this test?" If your HCP doesn't have an answer, then ask why you need the test. It's a great opportunity to open up a conversation. Many HCPs order tests out of habit, or sometimes, to cover themselves because they're afraid of being sued for malpractice. If you always ask how a test will affect your care, it will get your HCP thinking twice about what's ordered, and can save you time, aggravation, and money.

## BLOOD TESTS

### NURSE'S NOTE

Blood tests are ordered for one of three reasons: to screen for illnesses or risk factors for illness, to diagnose a condition, or to monitor therapy. For example, current guidelines call for measuring cholesterol and triglycerides in men at age 35 and women at age 45 to establish a baseline if there are no risk factors for cardiovascular disease. If risk factors are present, initial testing may be done anytime after age 20. This testing for blood fats is reasonable because if your levels are high, it puts you at risk for a heart attack, and treatment can bring the levels down.

If you have a rash, fatigue, and joint pain, your blood would be tested to see you have Lyme disease. A blood count can diagnose anemia, and by measuring hormone levels, you can learn if your thyroid is under or overactive. These are examples of diagnostic blood tests.

The third reason for blood testing is to monitor therapy. If you are taking anticoagulants (blood thinners), you'll need blood tests to make sure your blood doesn't take too long to clot or clot too soon. In other cases, instead of monitoring the effect of the medicine, blood tests can measure drug levels. Finally, if your cholesterol was a little high on screening, and you've undertaken a treatment plan to lower your cholesterol, a repeat test will see if your efforts have been successful.

### INSIDER INFO

#### What to ask your HCP about blood tests.

First, find out why you're having certain blood tests—to screen, diagnose, or monitor. Once you know the purpose, ask if there is anything you need to do so that the results will be as accurate as possible. For example, cholesterol levels are most accurate if you've been a teetotaler for at least 24 hours and if you've had nothing to eat and only water to drink for the 12 hours before the blood is drawn. Sometimes for convenience, if you need other blood tests, your HCP may order a screening cholesterol level, for example, even if you had lunch an hour before. If it's normal, you know you're okay because with proper preparation, it would have been even lower. If it's high, you can come back and repeat it under optimum conditions to see what the true level is.

If you're having a blood test to monitor treatment of some sort, ask if you should schedule the test at a special time—for example, a certain number of hours before or after you take your medicine.

**Learning about results.**
If it's a diagnostic test, before you have the blood drawn, discuss how you will get the results. If you've having an HIV test, you'll always get your results in person at an appointment with your HCP or another clinician at the testing center. Let your HCP know if you are particularly anxious about the results of any test and if you want a phone call or another appointment to discuss results in person. While your blood's being drawn, ask how long it will take for your HCP's office to get the results. Sometimes, tests need to be sent to a special laboratory, and results may take a couple of days. Otherwise, routine tests are all automatic today, and if anything is abnormal, the lab will call your HCP's office right away. You don't have to put your life on hold while you sit and wait a few days for the phone to ring if you speak up to clarify these matters before you go to the lab.

## NURSE'S WISDOM

For safety's sake, right after your blood is drawn, tell the person who drew it that you want to confirm that your name is spelled correctly and that labels with *your* name are on *your* blood tubes. Proper identification is critical, particularly if you're having a diagnostic test.

## NURSE'S WISDOM

### Preparing for medical imaging:

- Leave jewelry home. As much as we tease kids, these imaging machines don't care what you look like on the outside (and, no, you don't have to smile for your picture, either). Jewelry interferes with most imaging tests, so why take a chance that something might get lost? If you're driving in for a test on your lunch hour, take off your jewelry, and lock it and any other valuables in your glove compartment or trunk where they can't be seen through the windows. Ask how long the test will take when you schedule the appointment. Many medical imaging exams require that you drink a liquid called contrast, which will highlight certain structures. Or you may need an injection of contrast. Or, you may need to have some images taken, then wait and have more taken an hour later. Don't assume that everything is as quick as a chest X ray can be.

- Ask for written instructions if you need to do something to prepare for the exam. Most people are nervous when it comes to these things, and it's not a good idea to trust your memory with instructions given over the phone. If you miss a critical step, you may have to start from scratch on another day. You certainly want to avoid that! Instructions can be mailed, faxed, or e-mailed, or you can pick them up at the medical imaging department or your HCP's office. Some places even have all their instructions on a Web site.

- If your study requires a bowel prep (see p. 289) and/or contrast, it will take a while, and it will wear you out. Plan on taking it easy the rest of the day.

- Don't wear dark-colored socks (or pants) on a day you're having a barium study. If you have an, um, accident, everybody will know.

- Avoid wearing any clothing with metal because it will show up on the image. It's much easier to ask all patients to change into a gown so the technologists don't have to worry about a hidden metal bra hook, for example. But if you're going to be there for a while, or have arthritis, or are particularly sensitive to cold, there is no law that you must change. Here's how to be a fashion "do" for medical imaging. Women should avoid wearing a bra with metal hooks or an underwire. Instead, wear an elastic sports bra or none at all. Also wear regular underpants. Gentlemen, that means no boxers with snaps. For the next layer, a plain cotton T-shirt and pants with an elastic or drawstring (like sweatpants) work best. Avoid pants with zippers, or clips at the waist. And, since you will probably be freezing, top your outfit off with white cotton socks and a plain sweatshirt. Since I learned this trick about ten years ago, I haven't changed for an exam since. Now, you'll have to explain to the technologist that you know this insider trick. If you tell them there is no metal anywhere on your body, you should be okay. And, you'll be warmer, too.

## Preparing to take contrast or barium:

■ Ask the technologist for ideas if contrast or barium tastes nasty. Even if it makes you gag, you need to figure out a way to swallow the minimum amount—without vomiting—so you don't have to do it all over again. If you can get the liquid cold, the taste won't be as strong. You can also ask for a cup with an opaque cover—like a coffee cup—and a straw. You won't have to look at the stuff, and the straw will help direct it past your taste buds. I had to drink barium a few years ago, and I asked for it on the rocks in a to-go cup with a straw. It worked like a charm; otherwise, I never would have made it.

## Preparing for being cold:

■ Speak up! Medical imaging departments are cold, because the machines often generate a lot of heat. If you're working in the department and fully dressed, the chill isn't as apparent. If you're lying still on that rock hard metal table in a thin gown, you'll freeze. X rays, CT scans, and MRIs can be done through blankets, so be sure to ask for one (or a few) if you're chilly.

**Getting in position:**

■ Talk with your technologist about your comfort during an
X ray, MRI, or CT scan or ultrasound examination. Positioning is critical to get the right image—that is, for the part being
imagined. If you're having a study for your kidneys, and you
have a bad back, your legs do not have to be out straight on
that hard table. Ask for a pillow or wedge that you can rest
your legs on to take the stress off your lower back. Or, if the
technologist says you won't get in the way of the equipment,
just put your feet flat on the table with your knees bent if
you're lying on your back. If a technologist puts you in a position that's painful, speak up. This is particularly true for a
CT scan or MRI that takes a while. If you're in so much pain
you have to move during the imaging, they'll have to start
over. Work out a position you can tolerate before the imaging
starts. I have arthritis in my shoulders and when I had a CT
scan of my abdomen, I was supposed to put my arms over my
head for 15 minutes. I knew I couldn't keep my arms up for
that long, so we put our heads together to figure out how we
could get the images. There was nothing magical about my
hands being over my head, they just couldn't be at my sides.
By resting my arms on the frame of the scanner, I didn't have
to hold them up, and I didn't have to stretch them over my
head, which would have been very painful. We solved the
problem together and got great images. You can do that, too.

**Keeping yourself distracted:**

■ Ask for an open MRI if you have the slightest anxiety about the
walls closing in. When I had an MRI on those shoulders, they
asked me if I was claustrophobic and I said I wasn't. I wasn't
until they slid me in that tube! I had never been in such a closed
space. You can also bring your favorite CD. Today, all MRI
machines have sound systems and headphones (or speakers, if
they are scanning your head). Music can be very relaxing and
something familiar in a strange place is particularly nice.

- In the same vein, if you are having a long procedure, such as an angiogram or image-guided biopsy, bring your own headphones and tape or CD player so you can mentally be someplace else.
- Finally, if you are diabetic and had to fast for an imagining study, be sure you carry your own sugar with you in case your blood sugar level drops unexpectedly. The technologists will recognize the signs, but a ready source of sugar is not necessarily in every imaging room.

**Getting ready to leave:**
- If you've had to drink anything for a test, take a look in the mirror before you leave the department. The technologist may forget to tell you your lips are chalky white!
- Be sure to drink plenty of fluids for 24 hours after any medical imaging study that requires contrast to flush the contrast through your kidneys—whether you drank it or it was injected into your vein. Start with your first drink in the department before you leave.
- Before you leave the department, check with the technologist to see if there are any other special instructions you need to follow at home.
- If you're anxious about the results, ask if you can review the study with a radiologist before you leave the department.

# BOWEL PREP

## NURSE'S NOTE

Well, they may be able to transplant hearts and may soon be making clones of your favorite dog, but no one has come up with an easy way to clean out your intestines, or as we medical folks call it, a "bowel prep." This is a do-it-yourself procedure that has to happen before you can have some types of abdominal surgery, a colonoscopy, or certain medical imaging or X-ray examinations.

You may know when an HCP has not personally had the bowel prep experience when they're not particularly sympathetic to your plight. Having been there and done that myself, I have a lot of empathy and insight that someone with only "theoretical" knowledge may miss. Having been through bowel preps for laparoscopic surgery and medical imaging studies, I also know how critically important a good prep is. This is one of those situations in which "get it right the first time" applies—in spades.

## GET THEE TO THE ER

Call 911 for a ride if you've become seriously dehydrated from the laxatives you've taken for the bowel prep. Symptoms will include:

- Feeling like you're going to pass out when you stand up.
- Having very low blood pressure.
- Having a weak, rapid pulse.

## CALL YOUR HEALTH CARE PROVIDER

- If you're having watery, clear diarrhea and you have not completed all the steps of the bowel prep.
- If you think you are becoming dehydrated but are not so bad you need to call 911.

## INSIDER INFO

### The importance of a bowel prep.

Doing a proper bowel prep is very important for a number of reasons:

- If the bowel is empty during abdominal surgery, the risk of surgical infection goes way down.

- If the bowel (colon) is empty during a colonoscopy, the physician doing the procedure can see the lining of the colon and identify any abnormalities, especially polyps.
- If the bowel is empty, you'll get a higher quality X-ray examination of the kidneys, for example, because stool in the bowel can obscure the view of the kidneys on an X ray.

### Doing the two-step.

A bowel prep is a two-step process, although some people feel like they have to do the two-step to get to the bathroom in time once they've started the process. Seriously, make sure you have clear and ready access to a bathroom because you're likely to need it in a hurry. Mark off the calendar and plan to be home for the afternoon or evening before your procedure while you do the bowel prep. The two steps of the bowel prep are:

1. Taking medicines (laxatives) that help empty the bowel.

2. Restricting your diet so more stool won't form in the 12 hours before the test.

### Dynamite in a little box.

The goal of a bowel prep is to empty the bowel of stool. Note that key word empty. If you've gone to the bathroom eight times and all you produce is clear, watery diarrhea, congratulations! You have reached bowel prep nirvana.

This is a critical point. There are a number of steps in a standard bowel prep kit because each person responds differently. Me? I have a very sensitive intestine. The first time I did the prep, I had diarrhea like crazy after step one! I looked at all the other laxatives lined up on the counter and figured I would be completely dehydrated (or worse) if I used all of them. So I called my surgeon's office and talked with his nurse. She said, "Stop! No more!" And then she gave me instructions about how to, um, go from there.

People with less sensitive systems may need the laxative drink, pills, suppository and maybe even an enema chaser in the morning to achieve the desired results. The key is that once your bowel movements are clear and watery, you've emptied your bowel. If you've achieved this goal, check with your HCP or the medical imaging department before taking the rest of the items in the prep kit or on your instruction sheet. If your bowel movements are not clear and watery, keep following the prep instructions to, um, the bitter end.

### No gourmet meals, either.

A restricted diet is also critical to keep the bowel empty so that more stool does not form on one end of the intestine while you are get-

---

### ❓ Frequently Asked Questions

**Q.** *What are clear liquids?*

**A.** It's easy. These are fluids you can see through. Apple juice, yes; orange juice, no. Chicken broth, yes (nix the noodles); tomato soup, no. Milk? No way. Coffee? Black with sugar is okay. Tea is also a good choice (but no milk added). Alcohol? You're crazy. Granted, you can see through beer or vodka, but it's a bad idea to increase your urination when you're already on the verge of dehydration, and to consume alcohol on an empty stomach is really asking for trouble.

**Q.** *Is it true there's something special about red Jell-O and purple grape juice?*

**A.** Jell-O is also considered a clear liquid, but it has to be plain Jell-O without any fruits or other goodies added. Most bowel prep instructions caution against eating red Jell-O. That's because the red coloring can stain the lining of the intestine and look suspiciously like blood through a scope during a colonoscopy. If you're cleaning our your bowel for radiology (X ray), it's not an issue. But if someone is going to be looking at the inside of your intestine, it's best to stick with the lime or lemon flavor. Some HCPs also advise against purple grape juice or cranberry juice for the same reason.

ting rid of it on the other end. We call this a "clear liquid diet" because you should only consume liquids you can see through and not eat solid foods once you have started the laxative routine. The two together—emptying what is in the intestine plus limiting your food intake—are essential to a successful bowel prep.

After your procedure, your HCP will let you know when you can eat again. After X rays or colonoscopy, you can usually go back to a regular diet once you get home. If you've done a bowel prep before surgery, the procedure will determine when you'll be able to chow down again.

## LISTEN UP!

Certain people are at higher risk for dehydration and developing a low blood pressure during a bowel prep. You need to be extra careful if you:

- Take medicine every day to lower your blood pressure.
- Take medicine to lower your heart rate or control an abnormal rhythm.
- Are underweight.

Symptoms of low blood pressure include:

- Feeling lightheaded or woozy, particularly if you stand up fast from a sitting or lying position (or right after you go to the bathroom).
- Feeling very washed out.

Seniors and others who are not completely stable on their feet need to be particularly careful not to fall from wooziness caused by a lowered blood pressure or while rushing to get to the bathroom during a bowel prep.

# ENDOSCOPY

## NURSE'S NOTE

Endoscopy is a diagnostic procedure or screening test in which a physician looks inside one end of your gastrointestinal tract with a special instrument that has a lens, a bright light, and an opening through which instruments can be passed to collect tissue specimens. Upper endoscopy looks at the esophagus and stomach; on the other end, you can have a colonoscopy, in which the entire colon is examined, or a sigmoidoscopy, in which the lower part of the colon is examined.

These tests are becoming much easier to do because of advances in the technology and because we now have great drugs that will sedate you so that you won't remember anything, but you can follow instructions during the procedure and you won't be completely knocked out.

## CALL YOUR HEALTH CARE PROVIDER

- If you have bleeding or sharp abdominal pain after endoscopy (cramping after a colon exam is normal).

## INSIDER INFO

Apply the same standard to endoscopy as to any other tests—ask the HCP who thinks you need these tests how the results will change your care. Here's an example as to why: My father was hospitalized for pneumonia and had a reaction to the antibiotics that caused colon inflammation. He had bloody diarrhea for about two weeks and became anemic. A specialist was called in and said he needed to have a colonoscopy to evaluate the source of the bleeding. It was perfectly obvious to the rest of us that it was from the antibiotics, and even if there was a tumor, my father was way too sick for surgery or radiation or anything else. Bottom line? His treatment would not have changed one iota no matter what they found. I'll never forget how thrilled he was to tell the doctor no, he wasn't going to have another procedure.

## COMMON ENDOSCOPY EXAMINATIONS

### Sigmoidoscopy.

This procedure is sort of like the warm-up for the others. You still need to do the bowel prep, but most people don't need sedation for this procedure. The physician inserts a lighted tube into your rectum and then on into the lower third of your colon and examines the tissues for any abnormal growths. If a polyp is seen, it can be removed and sent to the lab for a biopsy. The procedure takes about 20 minutes, is done in the office, and once that tube is removed, you'll feel a whole lot better.

### Colonoscopy.

This is a more involved procedure, for which you will be sedated. In this procedure, a flexible lighted tube is inserted through the rectum to view the entire colon (a.k.a. the large intestine). To give you an idea of how much looking that entails, the tube is about six and a half feet long. You'll do a terrific bowel prep, and as with the sigmiodoscopy, any abnormal growths or tissue can be removed with very long, but tiny instruments and sent to the lab as a biopsy. Since you'll be sedated, consider the day lost. The procedure takes about an hour. Figure an hour or two recovery and then a nice, long nap when you get home.

### Upper endoscopy.

This is the same concept, but this time, the physician begins at the mouth and passes a slightly different lighted tube into the stomach. The good news? No bowel prep for this one. The better news? You get sedated for this, too. This procedure can be done to find out why someone needs antacids six days every week, to see how well an

> **? Frequently Asked Questions**
>
> **Q.** *Are there "results" for these tests?*
> **A.** If tissue was not removed and sent to the lab, the doctor can describe what he saw before you go home. You may not remember much of what was said, so a follow-up phone call a day or two later by the doctor can be very helpful. If biopsy specimens were sent to the lab, the doctor can tell you how long it takes to get results and whether he will call you or whether you should make an appointment to go over them in person.

ulcer is healing, or in an emergency, to identify a source of bleeding and stop it. It takes 30 to 60 minutes, with recovery just like the colonoscopy.

# SAME-DAY SURGERY

## NURSE'S NOTE

The number of one-day surgical procedures rises every year. As technology improves, the number of operations that can be done without an overnight stay in the hospital will continue to grow. Ten years ago, who would have thought that you could have your gallbladder taken out in the morning and sleep in your own bed that night?

## INSIDER INFO

Tell the surgeon (or the person in the office who sets up the operating room schedule) that you want to be the first case of the day. Granted, you have to get up shortly after you fall asleep and have someone drive you to the hospital in the dark before the sun comes up, but it's worth it. You can't eat or drink before surgery, so being first means you're not thinking about how hungry you are since you'll be in the operating room (OR) before you're even awake. And, if you're first into the OR, it's like the first appointment of the day at the dentist. They're not behind yet and you'll be home early.

Otherwise, you get assigned as a "TF" case, which means "to follow" other patients. You won't have a firm time for your surgery, and if there is an emergency or any type of delay, you'll be waiting around, starving and probably worrying, too. When I had cartilage removed from my knee, I was the last case the day before Thanksgiving, and didn't get home till 10 p.m.

Also, pick your anesthesiologist. That's right. You don't have to take potluck from the anesthesia department. When I had surgery, I asked my surgeon if it was his wife on the table, who would he want doing the anesthesia. For a friend, I called the secretary in the anesthesia office and asked who the nurses asked for when they had surgery. Either way, you'll get a good recommendation. If you're nervous about the procedure, and how you'll manage pain, or if you've never had anesthesia before, set up an appointment to meet and talk with the anesthesiologist before your surgery date. You'll be glad you did. It's great to see a familiar face, and it's smart to make friends with the person who has the really good drugs and controls your pain while you're there.

## POSTOPERATIVE PAIN

### NURSE'S NOTE

This is a brave new world for surgeons, but it can be scary when you're the patient. People are admitted to hospitals for nursing care, not more doctoring. So, instead of having someone like me checking on you regularly after your operation, when you go home the same day, you'll need to have a responsible adult with you for the first couple of days. (You'll have to negotiate whether or not nightly back rubs are part of your deal!)

I've had outpatient surgery twice, 14 years apart. Not only can I tell you things nurses know, but I can tell you the lessons I learned on the patient side of the bed about pain control.

## GET THEE TO THE ER

You'll get specific instructions depending on the type of surgery you had. However, any patient should get someone to call the surgeon and get a ride to the ER if:

- You have repeated vomiting and can't keep down any fluids.
- You have bleeding at your surgical site or stitches or staples have allowed the skin to open.
- You are in excruciating pain and the prescribed pain medicine isn't relieving it.

## CALL YOUR HEALTH CARE PROVIDER

- If you experience side effects from the medication that you can't tolerate.
- If pain is not well controlled with the prescribed medication.
- If you run a fever.
- If you're not sure about whether it's okay to do a certain activity.

## INSIDER INFO

Any nurse will tell you that taking pain medicine "as needed" after surgery is crazy. You got those good drugs, so take them as soon as you get home in your own bed. For the first 24 to 48 hours, take pain medicine on a schedule—every four to six hours as directed on the bottle. Don't wait till you're uncomfortable, because then you will continually be playing catch up. Stay head of the pain, don't let it get a jump on you.

Surgeons are learning more about pain management techniques all the time, both during surgical procedures and afterward. The problem is, some may forget to clue you in to what they did during the operation to reduce your pain, or they may tell you, but you may still be groggy and forget any discussion you may have had.

When I was in the recovery room after my knee operation, I expected it to hurt. Remarkably, it didn't! I was psyched. "This isn't so bad," I thought. When bedtime came, I wondered whether I should take my pain medicine or not. "I don't want to be all doped up," I thought. So I took some ibuprofen and went to bed.

At 2 a.m., I let out a scream because I was in excruciating pain. Nobody told us that the surgeon filled the knee with a long-acting anesthetic that would result in numbness for about 12 hours—or what would happen when it wore off.

### ? Frequently Asked Questions

Q. *Should I wait until I have pain before I take pain medication?*
A. No! That's not the most effective approach. Take the pain medicine every four to six hours regularly for the first 48 hours after surgery. If you wait until you are uncomfortable, or try to tough it out and take pain medicine sporadically, you'll have peaks of searing pain separated by periods of moderate relief. Ideally, you should have a constant level of pain control, which you'll achieve by regular dosing, not taking pills on an as-needed basis.

Q. *But won't I get addicted?*
A. Don't worry, you won't get addicted to pain medicine when you are taking it to relieve genuine pain after surgery. Funny how people don't worry about getting addicted to antibiotics for a sore throat or insulin for diabetes. If you need the medicine, take it.

Fourteen years later, I expected to be in pain and to have trouble getting out of bed after having small incisions made in my abdomen after my laparoscopy. Once more, I was amazed that I was able to get out of bed and go to the bathroom without help and essentially pain-free! Was it a miracle? You (or your companion, if you're too goofy from the sedation) need to ask if a long-acting local anesthetic was used at the end of the operation, and if so, the surgeon's best estimate of how long it will last. Then, do everything you can as long as you are stable to get out of that day surgery center and get comfy at home before the numbness goes away.

## TECHNICALLY SPEAKING . . .

For years, pain management specialists have been frustrated about the bad rap the word "narcotic" has taken. Technically, narcotics are pain medicines derived from opium or made synthetically. However, the general media has used the word "narcotic" to describe all kinds of illicit drugs from heroin to cocaine and PCP. Patients, understandably, have been nervous about taking "narcotics." So, in medical-speak, the terminology has changed to call these drugs, more appropriately, opioids. These medicines include many you are familiar with, such as morphine, Demerol, Vicodin, Percocet, Tylox, and codeine.

### Did You Know?

Nursing researchers studied 311 women who had gynecologic surgery. Patients who consciously relaxed their jaws and listened to music needed from 9% to 29% less pain medicine than patients who did nothing special. If you're coming home right after an operation, practice deep breathing and relaxation, and put on your favorite tunes; it will help you control your pain more effectively.

## NURSE'S WISDOM

Postoperative patients with good pain management do better. It's so simple, we learn it in Nursing 101. They get out of bed more often and walk around, which helps keep muscles strong and reduces blood pooling in the legs. Walking also helps combat the constipation that is associated with opioid pain medicine. And, if you're moving around, psychologically you'll feel better, which goes a long way toward speeding your recovery. Here are some suggestions for good pain management:

- Have prescription pain medicine ready to go. If you can, get the prescription ahead of time and get it filled before the surgery so your driver or companion doesn't have to figure out how to keep an eye on you and pick up a prescription at the same time on the day of surgery.
- The day before your surgery, prepare the room in which you'll be recovering. You might want to put fresh sheets on the bed, add an air freshener with a relaxing scent, and gather some extra pillows for comfort. Don't forget your pain-relieving tunes, too!
- Ask your nurse for a dose of pain medicine for the road. Receiving the medicine through IV is great if it won't make you so woozy that you'll be unsteady on your feet when you're trying to get out the door.
- Ask if you can safely take a dose of your pain pills as soon as you get home and settled in bed.

After the first 48 hours, based on your surgeon's instructions, you can usually reduce the prescription opioid pain medicine, or alternate doses with another type of pain medicine, the nonsteroidal anti-inflammatory drugs such as ibuprofen, naproxen, and ketoprofen. For example, take the prescription pain medicine at noon, then the ketoprofen at 3 p.m., another dose of the prescription medicine at 6 p.m. and so on.

## SELF-CARE

- Discuss a plan for pain management with your surgeon before your surgery. That way, you'll know what to expect, you'll be prepared, and you'll have more control over your care.
- Get postoperative care instructions (including the day and evening contact number of a care provider) before you go home. Make sure everything is in writing since you won't remember what anyone told you right after your surgery.
- Avoid a lot of activity—unless your surgeon says it's okay—the first 48 hours you're home. That means no lifting, bending, going up and down the stairs, and so forth.
- Be aware that pain medications can make you dizzy or woozy. Move with caution.
- Drink plenty of fluids and include fiber in your diet to help avoid a common side-effect of pain medication, which is constipation.

# APPENDIX: WEB RESOURCES

**General Health Resources**
**Healthfinder**
http://www.healthfinder.gov

**Medline Plus for Consumers**
http://www.nlm.nih.gov/medlineplus/

**I: TREATING SYMPTOMS**
Headache
**Medline Plus—Headache**
http://www.nlm.nih.gov/medlineplus/headache.html

**National Headache Foundation**
http://www.headaches.org/consumer/educationindex.html

**American Council for Headache Education**
http://www.achenet.org

Earache
**American Academy of Otolaryngology**—Head and Neck Surgery Patient Site
http://www.entnet.org/index2.cfm

**American Tinnitus Association**
http://www.ata.org

**National Institute for Occupational Safety and Health (NIOSH)**—Hearing Loss Prevention Site
http://www.cdc.gov/noish/topics/noise/

## Eye Irritation
**National Eye Institute of National Institutes of Health**
http://www.nei.nih.gov/health/index.htm

**American Optometric Association** (patient information)
http://www.aoanet.org/conditions/

**How to Protect and Care for Your Eyes**
http://www.amwa-doc.org/publications/WCHealthbook/eyesamwa-ch23.html

**State University of New York:** Using eye drops and ointments
http://www.sunyopt.edu/uoc/eyedrops.shtml

## Toothache or Mouth Pain
**National Oral Health Information Clearinghouse**
http://www.nohic.nidcr.nih.gov/links.html (for a list of links)
http://www.nohic.nidcr.nih.gov/searches.html (for a list of topics from the database)

**Dental Phobia Treatment Center**
http://www.dentalfear.net/index.html
While this is the site of a dentist in NYC, it provides a terrific explanation of dental phobia and what you should expect from your dentist.

## Back and Neck Pain
**All About Chiropractic Treatments**
http://www.spine-health.com/topics/conserv/chiro/feature/chirtro01.html

**Spine Health:** A comprehensive site including many points of view about back pain from orthopedic specialists, neurosurgeons, chiropractors, physical therapists and medical doctors
http://www.spine-health.com/index.html

**Good Body Mechanics**—How to move and lift while protecting your back
http://www.spineuniverse.com/displayarticle.php/article895. html

**Healthy Computing**
http://www.healthycomputing.com/office/setup/

## Bone, Muscle, and Joint Pain
**National Institute of Arthritis and Musculoskeletal and Skin Diseases**
http://www.naims.nih.gov/hi/topics/arthritis/oahandout.htm

**Fibromyalgia—Medline Plus** (provides links to approved sites)
http://www.nlm.nih.gov/medlineplus/fibromyalgia.html

**Carpal Tunnel Syndrome: American Physical Therapy Association**
http://www.apta.org/Consumer/ptandyourbody/carpaltunnel

**Chest Pain**
**Collapsed Lung: Pneumothorax**
http://www.pneumothorax.org

**Pleurisy from MedlinePlus**
http://www.nlm.nih.gov/medlineplus/ency/article/001371.htm

**Comparing Antacids from Drug Digest**
http://www.drugdigest.org/DD/Comparison/NewComparison/0,10621,8-14,00.html

**Digestive Diseases from the National Institutes of Health**
http://digestive.niddk.nih.gov/ddiseases/pubs/gerd/index.htm

**Weakness and Dizziness**
**Balance, Dizziness and You**
http://www.nidcd.nih.gov/health/balance/baldizz.asp

**Ménière Disease**
http://www.nlm.nih.gov/medlineplus/menieresdisease.html

**Cold and Cough**
**Questions and Answers about TB from the CDC**
http://www.cdc.gov/nchstp/tb/faqs/qa.htm

**Hold Your Own Against Cold & Flu**
http://www.fda.gov/fdac/features/2001/601_flu.html

**Cough Remedies from the Pharmacy at Wright State University**
http://www.wright.edu/admin/fredwhite/pharmacy/cough_r emedies.html

**Cough: The Merck Manual Online**
http://www.merck.com/pubs/mmanual/section6/chapter 63/63b.htm

**Smoking Cessation**
**Surgeon General's Smoking Cessation Guidelines**
http://www.surgeongeneral.gov/tobacco

**Medline Plus: Smoking Cessation**
http://www.nlm.nih.gov/medlineplus/smokingcessation.html

**American Lung Association Freedom from Smoking**
http://www.lungusa.org/ffs/overview.html

**Committed Quitters**
http://www.quit.com

**Nicoderm CQ**
http://nicodermcq.quit.com

**Stuffy or Runny Nose**
**American Rhinologic Society**
http://american-rhinologic.org and click on "Patient Information"

**Nasal Sprays:** How to use them correctly from American Academy of Family Physicians
http://familydoctor.org/handouts/104.html

**Nemours Foundation: What's a Booger?** For the kid in everyone (it does a great job explaining the nose's functions)
http://kidshealth.org/kid/talk/yucky/booger.html

**Sinus and Allergy Health Partnership**
http://www.sahp.org/index.html

**Sore Throat**
**American Academy of Family Physicians: Sore Throat**
http://familydoctor.org/handouts/687.html

**National Institutes of Health: Taking Care of Your Voice**
http://www.nidcd.nih.gov/health/voice/takingcare.asp

**Colgate University Student Health Services**
http://offices.colgate.edu/healthservices/hcsh_medication.html

**Fever**
**Medline Plus from the National Institutes of Health**
http://www.nlm.nih.gov/medlineplus/fever.html

**Abdominal Pain**
**The Medline Plus Medical Encyclopedia: Abdominal Pain**
http://www.nlm.nih.gov/medlineplus/ency/encyclopedia_A-Ag.htm

**Constipation and Diarrhea**
**Cleveland Clinic Department of Gastroenterology**
http://www.clevelandclinic.org/gastro/treat/diarrhea.htm

**North Carolina A&T State University,** *E.coli* **infection**
http://www.ces.ncsu.edu/teletip/scripts/1529.htm

## 2: TREATING AND PREVENTING INJURIES
### Sprains and Strains
**Sprains and Strains: National Library of Medicine**
http://www.nlm.nih.gov/medlineplus/sprainsandstrains.html

### Poison Control
**American Association of Poison Control Centers**
http://www.1-800-222-1222.info/poisonHelp.asp

**Home Cleaners** (what you can and cannot mix together)
http://www.practicalkitchen.com/hint_and_tips/homemade_cleaners.shtml

### Home Safety
**Consumer Product Safety Commission**
http://www.cpsc.gov

**Home Safety Council**
http://www.homesafetycouncil.org

**National Safety Council**
http://www.nsc.org

### Travel Safety
**Centers for Disease Control Traveler's Health Home Page**
http://www.cdc.gov/travel/index.htm

**Centers for Disease Control Travel in North America** (includes links to each state's health department)
http://www.cdc.gov/travel/namerica.htm

**Medical Information for Americans Traveling Abroad**
http://travel.state.gov/meidcal.html

**Transportation Security Administration** (airport security)
http://www.tsa.gov/public/display?theme=83

## 3: CHOOSING AND USING MEDICATIONS
### Resources to Share with Your Health Care Provider if You Can't Afford Prescription Medicine
http://www.helpingpatients.org

http://www.rxhope.com RxHope, 254 Mountain Avenue, Building B Suite 200 Hackettstown, NJ 07840 Telephone (908) 850-8004

http://www.rxassist.org

http://www.needymeds.com

**What You Must Know About Every Prescription**
American Pharmacists Association: Consumer Info
http://www.pharmacyandyou.org

American Society of Health-System Pharmacists
http://www.safemedication.com

Food and Drug Administration
http://ww.fda.gov

Information for Consumers
http://www.fda.gov/opacom/morecons.html

National Council on Patient Information and Education
http://www.bemedwise.com

**Antibiotic Alert**
Alliance Working for Antibiotic Resistance Education (AWARE)
http://www.aware.md

Barnard College Student Health Services: Antibiotics
http://www.barnard.columbia.edu/health/publications/antibiot.htm

Black Women's Health: Antibiotics
http://www.blackwomenshealth.com/antibiotics.htm

Centers for Disease Control: Antibiotic Resistance
http://www.cdc.gov/drugresistancecommunity

**Is It a Medication Allergy or a Side Effect?**
American Academy of Allergy, Asthma and Immunology
http://www.aaaai.org/patients/publicedmat/tips/adversereactions.stm

Discovery Health
http://health.discovery.com/diseaseandcond/encyclopedia/516.html

Medic Alert
http://www.medicalert.org

**Herbal Remedies and Supplements**
Do your homework. Here are some resources that will give you objective information:

National Center for Complementary and Alternative Medicine (part of the National Institutes of Health)
http://nccam.nih.gov/health/

**National Institutes of Health Office of Dietary Supplements Consumer Information Page**
http://ods.od.nih.gov/showpage.aspx?pageid=71

*PDR for Nutritional Supplements*
(http://www.pdrbookstore.com or your favorite bookstore)

*PDR for Herbal Medicines*
(http://www.pdrbookstore.com or your favorite bookstore) This one is on my bookshelf, and while it is quite technical, particularly on the botanical side, it has a very helpful cross-reference relating herbal medicines to symptoms and illnesses

**Alternative Medicine Foundation, Inc.**
http://www.amfoundation.org

**American Pharmaceutical Association—Herbal Medicines**
http://www.pharmacyandyou.org/healthinfo/herbal.html

FDA technical report on how to review evidence that does or does not support a health claim
http://vm.cfsan.fda.govms/SSAguide.html

**Federal Trade Commission: Dietary Supplements Advertising Guide**
Provides more than 30 examples of advertising claims that are and are not appropriate so you'll be able to recognize the difference

**MedlinePLUS Herbal Remedies**
http://www.nlm.nih.gov/medlineplus/herbalmedicine.html

**OTC Medications**
Type in the name of the medicine to learn more:

**PDR Consumer Health from Thomson Healthcare**
http://www.pdrhealth.com/drug_info/index.html

**RxList**
http://www.rxlist.com

**Safe Medication.com**
http://www.safemedication.com/meds/index.cfm

**Sites Where You Can Check for Drug Interactions**
**Drug Digest**
http://www.drugdigest.org/DD/Interaction/ChooseDrugs

**Drugs.com**
http://www.drugs.com/index.cfm?pageID=1150

On this page, read the terms, and if you agree, click "I agree" and you can go to the drug interaction page

**Drugstore.com**
http://www.drugstore.com/pharmacy/drugchecker/

The expert on interactions between medicines and grapefruit juice is at:
http://www.powernetdesign.com/grapefruit/

## 4: YOU AND YOUR HEALTH PROVIDER
### Choosing Your Primary Care Provider
**American Board of Medical Specialties**
http://www.abms.org

**American Medical Association Doctor Finder** (tells you board certification, medical school and where the doctor did training after medical school for AMA members and non-members)
http://www.ama-assn.org/aps/amahg.htm

### Getting the Most from Your Relationship with Your Health Care Providers
**The Resourceful Patient** Web-based patient empowerment!
http://www.resourcefulpatient.org/

**Common Sense Guide to Weight Management**
http://www.smartcalorie.com

Dr. Thomas Manger's web site that offers a wealth of information including a calculator that will give you nutritional information for your favorite recipe.

## 5: MEDICAL TESTS AND SAME-DAY SURGERY
### Bowel Prep
**National Institutes of Health: Sigmoidoscopy**
http://www.digestive.niddk.nih.gov/ddiseases/pubs/sigmoido scopy/index.htm

**Colonoscopy**
http://digestive.niddk.nih.gov/ddiseases/pubs/colonoscopy/index.htm

**Upper Endoscopy**
http://digestive.nddk.nih.gov/ddiseases/pubs/upperendoscopy/index.htm

# RESEARCH REFERENCES

**Oh! My Aching Head**
Holroyd KA, et al: Management of chronic tension-type headache with tricyclic antidepressant medication, stress management therapy, and their combination. *Journal of the American Medical Association* 2001;285:2208-2215.

**ED Study of Chest Pain**
Gaido, J: Gender bias in assessing patients with chest pain. 1999. New Brunswick, NJ.
Available at: http://www.stti.iupui.edu/VirginiaHendersonLibrary/Study FullView.aspx?SID=10933

**Sore Back: Better to Rest or Exercise?**
Powers C, Thayer P, Seymour RJ, Powers C, Thayer P, Seymour RJ: Effectiveness of exercise versus normal activity on acute low back pain: An integrative synthesis and meta-analysis. *Online Journal of Knowledge Synthesis for Nursing* 1999.

**Back Pain: What Works and What Doesn't?**
BMJ Publishing Group: Clinical Evidence Concise. Issue 8, Dec 2002; The Cochrane Library, Issue 3, 2003, Oxford: Update Software.

**Foods Can Trigger Asthma and Cough**
Emery NL, Vollmer WM, Buist AS, Osborne, ML: Self-reported food reactions and their associations with asthma. *Western Journal of Nursing Research* 1996;18(6):643-54.

**FAQ: Can vitamins and minerals cure a cold?**
Douglas RM, Chalker EB, Treacy B: Vitamin C for preventing and treating the common cold; Marshall I: Zinc for the common cold; Melchart D, et al: Echinacea for preventing and treating the common cold. All in: *The Cochrane Library*, 2, 2001. Oxford: Update Software. Available at: http://www.update-software.com/cochrane/

**Eat Thermometers and Accuracy**
Thomas KA, Savage MV, Brengelmann GL: Effect of facial cooling on tympanic temperature: *American Journal of Critical Care* 1997;6(1):46-51.

**Stress and Irritable Bowel Disorder**
Jarrett N, Heitkemper M, Cain KC, et al: The relationship between psychological distress and gastrointestinal symptoms in women with irritable bowel syndrome. *Nursing Research* 1998;47(3);154-61.

**Airport Security Screening Not Heart Stopping**
Kolb C, Schmieder S, Lehmann, et al: Do airport metal detectors interfere with implantable pacemakers of cardioverter-defibrillators? *Journal of the American College of Cardiology* 2003;41(11):2054-2059.

**Even if You Know the Ropes, You've Still Gotta Pull the Strings**
Rose LE, et al: The contexts of adherence for African Americans with high blood pressure. *Journal of Advanced Nursing* 2003;32(3):587-594.

**Better Supplement Your Knowledge First**
Taylor H, Leitman R eds: Widespread ignorance of regulation and labeling of vitamins, minerals and food supplements. *Harris Interactive Healthcare* 2002;2(23): December.

**Nurses Caring for Fewer Patients Means Better Outcomes**
Aiken LH et al: Hospital nursing staffing and patient mortality, nurse burnout, and job dissatisfaction. *Journal of the American Medical Association* 2002;288(16):1987-1993.
[please take note of where this very important research by nurses was published]

**Tune in Your Favorites, Tune Out Pain**
Good M et al: Relaxation and music reduce pain after gynecologic surgery. *Pain Management Nursing* 2002;3:61-70.

# INDEX